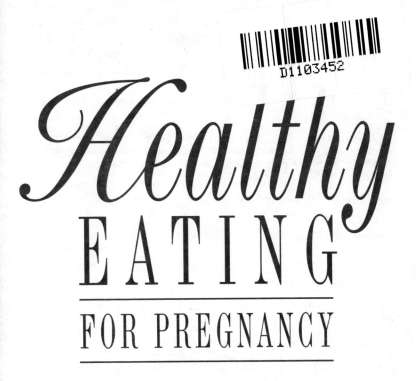

Healthy
EATING
FOR PREGNANCY

Wendy Doyle

TEACH YOURSELF BOOKS

I dedicate this book to Arthur and Margaret Wynn who have devoted so much time and effort working towards the prevention of disabilities in children and the wellbeing of mothers. They have been a source of inspiration and unfailing help to me and many others who share their ambitions.

Long-renowned as the authoritative source for self-guided learning – with more than 30 million copies sold worldwide – the *Teach Yourself* series includes over 200 titles in the fields of languages, crafts, hobbies, sports, and other leisure activities.

British Library Cataloguing in Publication Data

Doyle, Wendy
  Healthy Mum, Healthy Baby: Thinking about Pregnancy?
  I. Title
  613.04244

Library of Congress Catalog Card Number: on file

First published in UK 1995 by Hodder Headline Plc, 338 Euston Road, London NW1 3BH

First published in US 1997 by NTC Publishing Group
An imprint of NTC/Contemporary Publishing Company
4255 West Touhy Avenue, Lincolnwood (Chicago), Illinois 60646 – 1975 U.S.A.

Typeset by Wearset, Boldon, Tyne & Wear
Printed in Great Britain by Cox & Wyman Ltd, Reading, Berkshire.

Impression number 10 9 8 7 6 5 4 3
Year   1999 1998 1997

CONTENTS

ACKNOWLEDGEMENTS

I am grateful to my colleagues Somi Guha, Cheryl Louzado and Martin Leighfield at the Institute of Brain Chemistry and Human Nutrition for their help and advice in writing this book.

I would also like to thank Redmond Brown for his constant encouragement and guidance.

The information in this book is based on a review of current scientific literature. It is intended to be an information source, helping you make informed decisions; it is not under any circumstances to replace the advice of your doctor.

FOREWORD

The creation of a new life is a most precious act about which we are given much information. However, this is flawed information because it is highly selective. At schools we provide sex education for children. Yet little is taught about the requirements of the product of sex: of nourishing that new life during the critical period of early and very rapid development. Nothing is taught about the importance of health and nourishment of the mother and the father before pregnancy. The farmer knows the economic value of ensuring his animals are healthy and properly fed before conception. If these matters are demonstrably important for pigs, lambs and calves, how much more important they are for a new human life.

Why these matters are not taught is a puzzle. Possibly pregnancy is so commonplace that it is taken for granted by many. It may also have to do with the time it takes for advancing knowledge to become accepted in academic circles, get into the text books and then be incorporated into administrative thinking and practice. Until the 1980s, the means to study the way in which some 55 nutrients and 52 fatty acids in the diet relate to birth dimensions, such as low bodyweight, were not available: computers have changed that.

Wendy Doyle's book sets out the physiological and nutritional principles and provides the material that medical practitioners, dieticians, midwives, health visitors and students need. It is written in a readily accessible style which should make it compulsory reading for anyone who is planning to have a child.

That pregnancy must not be taken for granted is demonstrated by the fact that we have 54,000 low-birthweight babies born each year in the UK. The incidence of severe disorders such as mental retardation, deafness, blindness, cerebral palsy and autism is some thirty times greater in very-low-birthweight babies. The incidence of low birthweight has remained unchanged over the last 30 years but disorders amongst low-birthweight babies has trebled despite the advances in obstetrics and paediatrics. There is also increasing evidence that low birthweight is associated with risk of heart disease, stroke and diabetes in later life.

Wendy Doyle began her work on nutrition and pregnancy in 1978 in collaboration with myself and Dr Bernard Laurence during the time he was Secretary to the British Paediatric Association. Since then she has published many papers describing the relationship between maternal nutrition and pregnancy outcome. So she brings a wealth of experience and new knowledge to bear in her book.

Two important conclusions emerge from her work: First, that nutrient intakes correlate with birthweight independent of smoking or alcohol up to but not above 3270 g (7.2 lb). The importance of this conclusion lies in the fact that the risk is not confined to babies born below the usual demarcation point of low birthweight (2500 g or 5.5 lb) but is linked to all those in the lower range of birthweights. This is the same range where Wendy has shown that maternal nutrition matters to birthweight. The second conclusion is that the diet of the mother at or about the time of conception is of greater significance to pregnancy outcome than her diet during the latter part of pregnancy.

These conclusions are totally logical. In any field of endeavour, getting things right at the start is the key to success. Wendy Doyle's book will, I hope, be read by professionals and lay people alike, and will, therefore, contribute to a greater understanding of the need for good health in parents and their future children.

Professor Michael A. Crawford CIBiol, FIBiol

1

THE BEGINNING

For a woman, the birth of her first child is both an end and a beginning: it is the end of her pregnancy and the beginning of motherhood. The start of motherhood and the life of her child is a moment to be thought about and planned very carefully.

There is perhaps no greater happiness than a child delivered whole and healthy into the world. It is an event that many of us take for granted; but what if the baby is not born healthy? What if the baby is born with a disability that may affect the rest of his or her life? All mothers, at some time, have concerns such as these.

Thanks to nature and the medical profession, the vast majority of births happen successfully; but we cannot afford to leave all things to nature, or hope that a doctor can always correct something that has gone wrong. All parents share the responsibility to do what they can to ensure the best possible conditions and environment exist to enable their baby to be born healthy.

No one would buy a house without careful consideration and planning, so why is it not commonplace to plan seriously, having a baby? Why do we not make sure that we are as healthy as possible before bringing a new life into the world – a life that will affect the rest of our lives, and those of our extended families?

It is a great credit to the medical profession, as well as to nature, that so many births happen successfully. Due to their skill, most of the 50,000 babies who are born each year in the UK weighing less than $5\frac{1}{2}$ lb – the official demarcation point for low birthweight – will survive. Many of these babies will, however, spend the first days or weeks of their life in special incubators in intensive care. The parents can do no more than stand by and observe their baby, unable to pick it up, to cuddle it, and make the basic bonding contact so necessary in early development.

The ability to save the lives of babies who even twenty years ago may have died carries problems in its wake. Many low-birthweight babies are sadly left with some degree of handicap. A typical problem is *cerebral palsy*, a devastating disease leading in severe cases to paralysis and mental retardation. Tragically, with the increased survival of low-birthweight babies, the incidence of cerebral palsy has increased threefold since the 1960s (Pharoah et al., 1990).

Another disease, *spina bifida*, often referred to by the medical profession as a *neural tube defect*, claims 400 severely handicapped babies each year in the UK. It is now known that this disease is largely preventable by nutritional intervention around the time of conception.

The causes of low birthweight, which increases the risk of handicap to your baby, include poor diet, especially around the time of conception, smoking, and other environmental factors.

─────── Before the beginning ───────

You will be hoping for a safe and successful pregnancy, at the end of which you will deliver an infant whose physical and mental potential is not impaired. To give you and your baby every chance of a successful outcome, you need to assess your lifestyle and make thoughtful preparations before conception.

At the stage where your baby is still in the planning stage, time is on your side. During this time before pregnancy, you and your partner should examine your health, diet and lifestyle. For there is much evidence that good health at the time of conception has a critical role to play in the health of your baby. These foundations, or lack of them, are important not only for your baby's survival at birth, but will also have an impact during its formative years and on its health in adult life.

The fact that your health at the time of conception is of such importance to the health of your baby is perhaps more understandable if you consider the events that take place in the womb during the first few weeks after creation.

We all start life as a single cell, a result of the fusion of male *sperm* and female egg. That one cell in turn multiplies into six billion cells within the first ten weeks of pregnancy. These cells, laid down in the first few weeks of pregnancy, contain the structural foundations of a child's future body and much of this will have occurred before most mothers-to-be know they are pregnant.

– The changing profile of an embryo –

3 WEEKS AFTER CONCEIVING

Development has already begun of:

- the heart
- blood vessels
- the brain and spinal cord

4 TO 8 WEEKS AFTER CONCEIVING

- arms and legs begin to develop
- rapid brain growth occurs
- eyes and nose are recognisable
- hands form
- elbows and wrists are identifiable
- ears are visible
- eye colour is determined
- the heart begins to beat
- fingers and toes are visible
- eyes open and lids form
- the lungs, kidneys and liver are developing
- the genitalia appear

At the end of eight weeks, the baby already looks human although it only measures about 1 inch (2·5 cm) in length. Not surprisingly, with all this very rapid development taking place, there is a very high requirement for the basic nutrients necessary for body growth including protein, essential fatty acids, vitamins and minerals.

The *placenta* (the link between mother and baby, which supplies nutrients and oxygen) only starts to work in the second month, before which the embryo, and before that the developing *follicles* in the *ovary*, are dependent on the nutrients circulating in the mother's blood and are not protected from deficiencies.

Laying the foundations of a house without the correct amount of materials and preparation would be folly. It does not matter how big a house you build; if any faults are present when the foundations are laid, it is almost impossible to correct those faults later. In a similar way, any defects in the early stages of development of a baby are usually permanent and can seldom be rectified.

Professor David Barker of Southampton University suggests that the relative health of our organs and systems, such as the heart and *vascular* (veins and arteries) system, are determined at very specific times during embryonic and *fetal* growth. These critical moments of development often represent a very brief window of time and once passed can never be recaptured.

Repeated studies have suggested that a mother's diet at the time she conceives is critical to the health and development of her baby. This is borne out by experiments with animals, where low birthweight and growth retardation are induced by depriving the mother of essential nutrients before and immediately after mating. This is also consistent with the reproductive cycle of animals in their own habitat, where mating is naturally timed to coincide with the maximum availability of food. As with animals, it seems increasingly likely that even subtle vitamin and mineral deficiencies have an adverse effect on development in the womb. As a low-birthweight child grows up, organs that may have already been compromised during fetal development are prone to failure, when following the lifestyles most of us lead, with little exercise, poor diet, smoking, stress and so on.

We now know more about the effects of our lifestyle and eating habits on pregnancy than ever before. We also know more about how fertility, conception and pregnancy are vulnerable not only to nutritional deficiencies but also to infections, toxic substances and inherited diseases.

In this book I hope to describe the potential risk factors so that parents-to-be can examine their lifestyles and make the changes they feel are appropriate to them.

──────── Why prepare? ────────

Preparing for conception is not a new idea. The association between nutrition and a healthy outcome of pregnancy goes back hundreds of years. In 1608 a French midwife called Louyse Bourgeois published a book in which she claimed that poor prenatal nutrition could lead to premature birth. What is new is the breadth and depth of evidence that has emerged from scientific and medical research about how the health and nutritional status of the parents is important, particularly around the time of conception.

Most women, if asked about the birth of their child, will say 'as long as it's healthy'. This usually overshadows any other considerations such as the sex of the baby or worries about labour. Most women are unaware of the critical significance of the weeks before the pregnancy is confirmed. Obstetrician Dr Hamish Sutherland wrote in the *Lancet*:

> ❦ Too many women make (their) first antenatal visit with the pregnancy already compromised or at risk from smoking, inappropriate nutrition, ingestion of a variety of pharmaceutical preparations . . . , genito-urinary infection, Anaemia, and poor dental hygiene. All too frequently Cervical Cytology and Rubella immunity status are unknown. ❦

Of course, most women know they are pregnant some time before their first visit to the antenatal clinic but even then, they may be five or six weeks into their pregnancy before they can act on that knowledge. Most problems in early development originate between three and eight weeks after conception.

Critical periods in human development

A healthy pregnancy starts before conception with healthy parents. In the woman, low levels of the two most important reproductive *hormones* (oestradiol and progesterone) are associated with poor outcome of pregnancy as well as with early miscarriage. If these hormone levels are low, but not low enough to cause infertility, ovulation (the release of an egg from the ovary) is slowed down and the immature egg may be smaller in size than normal. This slow- down is associated with retarded fetal growth and birth abnormalities. Low levels of these reproductive hormones can be induced simply by restricting your diet (Pirke et al., 1985). Your nutritional status is therefore very important even before your last period.

A man's biological contribution to pregnancy may end at conception but it is nonetheless a crucial one. Damage to sperm is a frequent cause of infertility, miscarriage and other consequences. This damage to sperm can result from smoking, alcohol, exposure to radiation and to some chemicals and drugs, poor nutrition, and infections such as influenza, measles or mumps. The time it takes to eliminate damaged sperm can vary, but usually sperm get a clean bill of health four months after exposure to the damaging substance.

After conception, there are three very important developmental stages during pregnancy:

Stage 1 The 'pre-embryonic' stage lasts for three weeks, starting with the moment of fertilisation and continuing after implantation in the womb, until the embryo begins to grow. During the two weeks following fertilisation, the 'zygote', or fertilized egg, divides many times. It does not increase in size much at this time, but it is a critical period developmentally and a time when both mother and child will benefit from the best possible supply of nutrients because cell division is a nutrient-driven process.

Stage 2 The 'embryonic' stage begins at the fourth week after conception and lasts until the eighth week. Physical changes to the embryo take place during this stage of very rapid cell division, when all the major organs begin to form.

Stage 3 From the ninth week the embryo is termed a fetus with its own complete central nervous system and a beating heart. The fetus continues to grow and develop until birth.

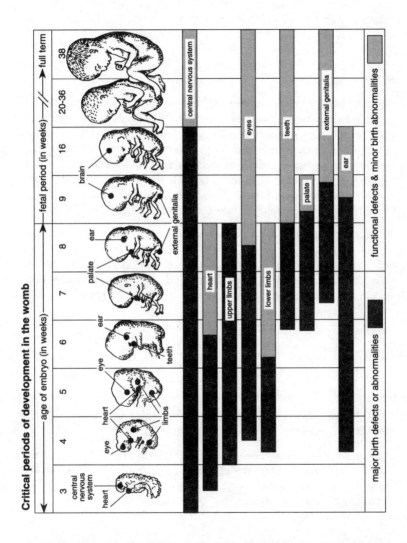

The critical periods in human development. Dark shading denotes highly sensitive periods when major defects may be produced. Dotted shading indicates stages that are less sensitive to damaging agents when minor defects may be induced.

The most critical phase in the development of the embryo, or in the growth of a particular organ, is during its time of rapid cell division. This is because cells are generally more susceptible to damage when dividing. Each organ is most dependent on an adequate supply of nutrients during its own intensive period of growth. For example, the heart and brain are well developed at 14 weeks, while the critical period of growth for the lungs is not until 10 weeks later. This means that poor nutrition early in pregnancy may affect the heart and brain, while malnourishment later in pregnancy is more likely to affect development of the lungs.

Stage 2, from week 3 to week 8, is the period of greatest environmental sensitivity for the developing baby. During this period the process of cell organisation takes place and the foundations of the major organs are being laid. Any adversity at this time, whether nutrition-, infection- or drug-associated, can compromise the development of the baby. If embryonic cell division is slowed down, there is an increased risk of congenital malformations due to growth being out of step (Eckhert and Hurley, 1977).

Events during a critical period of development can take place only at that time and no other. Whatever nutrients are needed at the time must be supplied on time if the developing organ is to reach its full potential. If development is curbed during a critical period, recovery is not possible later. Early malnutrition can have irreversible effects.

————— Low birthweight —————

Low birthweight is classified as a baby weighing less than 2500 g or $5\frac{1}{2}$ lb at birth whether born prematurely or full term.

Approximately 50,000 low-birthweight babies are born in the UK each year. Despite advances in obstetric care, the incidence of low birthweight has proved very resistant to change. There is still approximately the same number of low-birthweight babies born in the UK today as there was in the 1950s.

It is generally agreed that low birthweight is the most practical measure of a poor pregnancy outcome because it is a major determinant of infant mortality. Low birthweight infants are also at greater risk of illness in general. They are three times more likely to suffer adverse neurological (brain and central nervous system) developments, and the risk of damage increases with decreasing birthweight. The incidence of severe neurological disorders increases from less than 1 per cent in babies weighing between 3500 and 4500 g (7 lb 11 oz and 9 lb 14 oz) to over 20 per cent in the very-low-birthweight group weighing 1500 g (3 lb 5 oz) or below (Office of Population, Censuses and Surveys, 1988). These disorders include cerebral palsy, mental retardation, blindness, deafness, epilepsy and autism.

Low-birthweight infants are also thought to be more susceptible to a wide range of other conditions such as respiratory infections, learning disorders and behavioural problems (Institute of Medicine, 1985). In a study of over nine hundred very-low-birthweight babies born in Scotland, almost a third had died by the age of four, 47 had cerebral palsy, 11 were deaf and 7 were blind. Of the remaining children, almost half had poor attention spans and overall they performed poorly on visual recognition, numeric skills and verbal comprehension (Scottish Low Birthweight Study, 1992).

Low birthweight and poor fetal growth may also be associated with chronic illness in later life, particularly from heart disease. Professor Barker and his colleagues suggest that cardiovascular disease originates through programming of the body's physiology early in fetal life (Barker et al., 1993).

Birthweight is therefore important not just to survival, but also in allowing individuals to reach their potential in terms of physical and intellectual development and general health in later life.

Low birthweight and congenital abnormalities

Abnormalities at birth usually have one of two causes: genetic or environmental.

Genetic influences may give rise to an inherited alteration of the *chromosomes* that carry genetic information. These family-inherited abnormalities cannot be prevented, although their impact may be reduced with the help of genetic counselling.

Environmental influences include infections such as German measles, dangerous drugs, nutritional deficiencies such as a lack of certain vitamins, or physical injuries such as those caused by radiation and X-rays. Some of these are identifiable and therefore can be avoided.

In recent years there has been a dramatic decline in infant mortality rates. More and more premature babies now survive at lower and lower weights, when 20 years ago they would unquestionably have died. Sadly, there is a down-side to this; the increase in survival rates of these very small babies has been associated with an increase in the rates of handicapped children surviving. A study in Liverpool reported a threefold increase in the number of low-birthweight babies born with cerebral palsy since 1976. The same trends are being seen in other countries such as Sweden and Australia.

Causes of low birthweight

Low birthweight may be due either to the baby being born pre-term (less than 37 weeks), or it may be born at term but be small as a consequence of retarded growth during fetal life. In the developed world, approximately two-thirds of all low-birthweight babies are pre-term and one-third are growth-retarded (World Health Organisation, 1980).

Despite advances in obstetrics and maternal/fetal medicine, our understanding of the causes of pre-term birth and fetal growth retardation is limited. Genetic factors are thought to explain 25 to 35 per cent of low birthweight, and environmental influences the remainder (Metcoff, 1981; Fedrick and Adelstein, 1978). Poor maternal nutrition is likely to be a major environmental 'cause' of retarded growth. If this is so, a substantial proportion of cases of low birthweight is preventable.

In reality, there are probably many causes which result in a baby being born with a low birthweight, and much information has been gathered on so-called 'risk factors'. There is a variety of risk factors that are consistently linked to low birthweight. The importance of each factor for an individual cannot easily be calculated, and should be viewed as a relatively crude indicator of risk. Their presence in an individual woman indicates an increased chance of having a poor pregnancy outcome, and they have a cumulative effect – the more factors that apply to an individual, the greater the overall risk of a disappointing pregnancy outcome.

—— Checklist for self-assessment ——

The following list is to help you to examine your own environmental and genetic background for possible risk factors that could influence your pregnancy. No one can guarantee a healthy baby, but you can increase your chances of a healthy outcome if you try to:

- Eat a healthy diet
- Stop smoking
- Drink alcohol sparingly, if at all
- Be a good weight for pregnancy
- Avoid inappropriate drugs and medicines
- Check your immunity to rubella
- Attend to known health problems
- Avoid environmental hazards, such as X-rays and chemicals
- Practise food hygiene
- Take some form of exercise
- Allow time between pregnancies
- Take 400 mcg folic acid supplement daily
- Stop eating liver

After reading this book and understanding the reasons why changes might be beneficial, you and your partner can tick off any modifications you could make. Try to make these changes three to six months before stopping contraception.

2

A HEALTHY DIET

A recent conference on 'The Influence of Maternal Nutrition on Pregnancy Outcome' concluded:

> ❦ Prevention of a significant proportion of birth defects low-birthweight babies, and Sudden Infant Death Syndrome has been shown to be possible by enhancement of the micronutrient status of women of childbearing potential and those already pregnant. Further reduction in the risk of adverse pregnancy outcomes could be achieved with pre-pregnancy counselling to avoid cigarette smoking, alcoholic drinks, illicit drugs, low calorie dieting, and other unhealthy habits. Improved pre-pregnancy medical care, with a strong emphasis on the nutritional needs of the Embryo, Fetus, Neonate, and mother is clearly warranted ... the consequences include the obvious reduction in human misery as well as a significant decrease in medical expenses. ❧

This, and results from many other studies, draw the conclusion that diet plays a central part in pre-pregnancy planning. For that reason this book will pay a great deal of attention to the subject of healthy eating.

Importance of early nutrition

There is no doubt that your pre-pregnancy nutrition plays a vital part in the early development of your baby.

Two illustrations of this are the well-documented relationship of iodine and folic acid in aiding a healthy pregnancy. These two nutrients are highlighted here to illustrate the success of altering your diet prior to pregnancy, but it must be remembered that iodine and folic acid are only two elements of a broad band of nutrients that are vital for enhancing the environment within the womb.

Iodine

The story of iodine was one of the first clues to the importance of nutrition in relation to pregnancy, especially around the time you conceive. It highlights how healthy development of your baby can be dependent on a single nutrient being present in adequate amounts.

Iodine deficiency was identified in British Columbia in the early 1920s, when doctors noticed wide discrepancies in the numbers of mentally retarded children found amongst inland settlers' children when compared to the coastal Indians. Dietary differences were also observed between these two groups of people. The coastal Indians, whose diet was richer in iodine due to the amount of fish and seafood they ate, had a dramatically reduced incidence of retarded children (*cretinism*). Through these early studies it was found that by the introduction of iodine into the pre-pregnant woman's diet this type of embryo malformation could be avoided.

Cretinism can be prevented simply by correcting iodine deficiency before and during the first three months of your pregnancy. Today, cretinism should have been totally eradicated by dietary intervention. Sadly, in parts of the world, where iodised salt or other means of iodine supplementation could save babies and their families from the dreadful consequences of cretinism, it remains a serious problem.

Fortunately, iodine deficiency in Britain is rare because iodine is found in fish and is also present in our soil, except in small geographical pockets such as in Derbyshire and the deep valleys of the Pennines, Cotswolds and Mendips. In earlier times, iodine deficiency in these areas led to a high incidence of *goitre* (often referred to as Derbyshire Neck). Today, dietary diversification, made possible by improved distribution of food, has corrected any underlying local deficiencies.

Folic acid

The most common major fetal malformations in the UK are those of the central nervous system, referred to collectively as *neural tube defects*. These defects, which include *spina bifida* and *anencephaly*, occur if the brain and/or the spinal cord fail to develop correctly around four to six weeks after conceiving. About 400 babies are born severely disabled with spina bifida each year in the UK (DoH, 1992). Children born with neural tube defects often die, and those that survive have a wide range of physical disabilities and face a life of severe handicap.

An illustration of the relationship between pre-pregnancy nutrition and a successful pregnancy can be found in the protective effects of one of the B vitamins – folic acid. In 1991, the Medical Research Council published the results of their study on the use of folic acid supplementation (Wald et al., 1991). This study found a positive relationship between folic acid and the prevention of neural tube defects. The study looked at 1817 women who had previously had a baby with a neural tube defect, and was carried out in seven countries. These women were at high risk of having another damaged baby in their subsequent pregnancies. Fifty per cent of the women were prescribed folic acid supplementation in the months prior to conceiving and the early weeks of pregnancy. The trial showed that the mothers who were given folic acid around the time they conceived had a low risk of having another damaged baby.

The evidence was so overwhelming that the Department of Health now recommends that any woman who is planning to become, or could become, pregnant should take a supplement of 400 mcg a day and should be encouraged to choose foods that are rich in folic acid such as leafy green vegetables, oranges, fortified bread and breakfast cereals.

Folic acid, because of its importance to people living in this country, is discussed in more detail later in this book (see page 27).

Recommended intakes

Folic acid and iodine are not the only nutrients to concentrate on, and this chapter will consider the practical issues in following healthy eating recommendations when preparing for pregnancy. In the days before the nutritional constituents of food were known, dietary requirements were based on the amount of food eaten by healthy people. The daily ration for Roman soldiers was said to be one *librum*, which was equivalent to 1 lb of wheat. Today, we take a more scientific approach. Nutrient targets are set for men, women and children in different age-groups, also for women during pregnancy and while breast-feeding. This is more scientific, but it is difficult to translate these recommended nutrient levels into everyday food intake. For instance, the recommended intake of calcium, which will meet the requirements of almost all pre-pregnant women, is 700 mg a day; this prompts the question: which foods do I get this from, and how much of these foods do I need to eat to acquire it? This question applies to all nutrients for which there are published recommendations (DoH, 1991). Help with these questions is necessary, as even those trained in nutrition often find it difficult to say with certainty that their own food intakes meet the recommended levels for all essential nutrients.

Many of us think we have a healthy diet but a government survey on the diets of British adults suggests that few of us meet all the recommendations (Gregory et al., 1990). The following section will briefly discuss *energy* (calories), the *'macro' nutrients* which are the energy-providing nutrients, protein, fat and carbohydrate and the *'micro' nutrients*, that is vitamins and minerals, paying particular attention to those considered important to preparing for pregnancy.

Energy

Energy is obtained from food through the intake of protein, fat and carbohydrate. Energy-yielding nutrients are vital to life, for without continual replenishment of energy you could not survive.

Some people perceive 'energy' as being good because we all need energy, but 'calories' as being bad because too many mean putting on weight. In reality, they mean the same thing – a calorie is simply a measure of energy.

This measure of energy, a *calorie* (sometimes called *kilocalorie* or *kcalorie*) is scientifically defined as the amount of energy necessary to raise the temperature of 1 kg of water by 1 degree centigrade. However useful this definition is to scientists, it is of little value to the average person cooking a meal; but in practical terms, it takes about 20 kcalories to boil a cup of water – this amount of energy is equivalent to one teaspoon of sugar.

Calories are essentially the vehicle of energy. It is the foods from which we obtain these calories that dictate the quality of our diet. Vegetables, fruit, cereals, lean meat, fish and dairy foods are rich in a wide spectrum of essential nutrients. Other foods containing high amounts of sugar and fat often hidden in everyday foods, have few or no essential nutrients. These are commonly called 'empty' calories. Having sufficient kcalories (energy) is important but cannot be viewed in isolation from the sources from which it was obtained.

The following examples illustrate the wide variation of nutrients obtained from a portion of two different snacks of equal kcalorie content:

	Rich Tea biscuits (5 biscuits)	Branflakes & low fat milk (1 portion)
Energy (kcal)	**200**	**200**
Protein (g)	2.9	8.4
Fibre (g)	0.7	6.5
Vitamin B1 (mg)	0.06	0.5
Vitamin B2 (mg)	0.04	0.8
Vitamin B3 (mg)	0.7	7.6
Vitamin B6 (mg)	0.0	1.3
Folic acid (mcg)	5.7	130
Calcium (mg)	53	145
Iron (mg)	0.9	10.1
Zinc (mg)	0.3	2.1
Magnesium (mg)	7.5	77

Data/information from The Composition of Foods, 5th ed. (1991) is reproduced with the permission of the Royal Society of Chemistry and the Controller of Her Majesty's Stationery Office

Energy requirements

Individual calorie requirements vary enormously. Most of us will have friends who seem to eat enormous amounts of food and not put on weight. Conversely, other less fortunate people seem to put on weight while eating very little.

Energy requirements are determined largely by the amount of energy you use, your basal metabolic rate and any special energy needs, such as growth, pregnancy and breast-feeding. Your basal metabolic rate is simply the rate at which your body uses energy while at complete rest. This will include energy to maintain your body temperature and other normal functions such as heartbeat, breathing and many other involuntary functions such as brain function and muscle tone. If your energy intake from food is greater than your total energy use, the balance will be turned into fat and stored as an energy reserve. Assuming your weight is right for your height (see Appendix 2), the ideal is to balance your energy intake and energy output.

Energy balance will, in general, be indicated for an individual by their weight. If your weight is stable (e.g. varies less than a few pounds either way over a six-month period) and appropriate for your height (see Appendix), your calorie intake is correct for your needs.

'Input'   'Output'

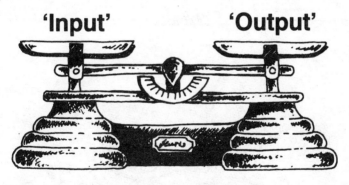

Try to balance your energy input and your energy output

The Department of Health recommends that the energy requirement for women who are not pregnant (aged 19–50 years) is 1940 kcal a day. Teenage girls require a little more (2110 kcal) to satisfy their growth requirements. During pregnancy, an increase of 200 kcal per day is recommended for the last trimester (weeks 27 to 40) of pregnancy only.

A low calorie intake makes it very difficult to meet all your nutritional requirements. On the other hand, it is quite possible to eat sufficient in terms of calories but to have a low intake of vitamins and minerals if you choose foods with a low nutrient density (i.e. the proverbial 'junk foods', high in fat and/or sugar but low in vitamins and minerals).

Nutrient density is a term used by nutritionists to express the nutrient quality of a food or a person's total food intake. This is judged by the amount of individual vitamins and minerals in a fixed number of calories, for example, in 1000 kcal.

AN EXAMPLE OF NUTRIENT DENSITY

Food	No. of kcalories	Vitamin B3 (niacin) grams
Bread, wholemeal	1000	19.1
Bread, white	1000	7.2
Biscuit	1000	0.8
Sugar	1000	trace

Data/information from The Composition of Foods, 5th ed. (1991) is reproduced with the permission of the Royal Society of Chemistry and the Controller of Her Majesty's Stationery Office

Protein

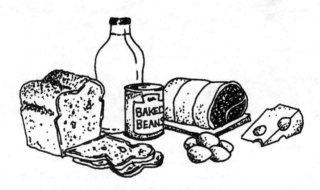

In the past, almost to the exclusion of other nutrients, protein was given the central nutritional role in relation to pregnancy because of the part it plays in the growth of new tissue. However, growth is a complex process that requires more than just an adequate amount of protein. While protein is essential for tissue growth, foods also high in protein are 'carriers' of some important minerals and trace elements including iron and zinc.

The diet of most people living in the Western world contains more protein than they need and protein not required for tissue growth is used for energy or converted into fat. The average intake of protein for women in the UK is 62 g a day, while the estimated average requirement is 36 g, and 45 g a day will meet the needs of almost all women. An extra 6 g a day is required to meet the needs of pregnancy.

The primary sources of protein in our diet come from three main food types – meat and meat products (36 per cent), bread and cereal products (23 per cent) and dairy foods and eggs (21 per cent).

Protein is made up of amino acids. Eight of these are 'essential' amino acids which the human body cannot make, so they must be obtained from your diet. They are all readily available from animal sources of protein including fish, but vegans and strict vegetarians must eat a mixture of pulses, nuts and cereal foods to help maintain the balance of essential amino acids. Plant sources of protein are listed below:

PLANT SOURCES OF PROTEIN

		Portion size	Grams of protein
Vegetables	Beans, baked	small can/150 g	7.8
	Beans, red kidney, tinned	3 tbs/105 g	7.2
	Peas, frozen	3 tbs/90 g	6.0
	Spinach, boiled	avg ptn/90 g	2.0
	Sweetcorn, kernels	3 tbs/90 g	2.6
Nuts	Peanuts	small bag/25 g	6.1
	Hazelnuts	1 oz/25 g	3.5
	Peanut butter	1 oz/25 g	5.6
Meat substitutes			
	Quorn	3 oz/85 g	10.0
	Tofu	3 oz/85 g	12.0
Bread	Bread, wholemeal	2 slices/70 g	6.4
Pasta	Spaghetti, white, boiled	8 oz/220 g	7.9
Rice	White or brown, boiled	6 oz/170 g	4.4

Data/information from The Composition of Foods, 5th ed. (1991) is reproduced with the permission of the Royal Society of Chemistry and the Controller of Her Majesty's Stationery Office

Fat

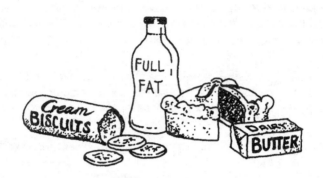

Most of us living in the Western world eat more fat and saturated fat than is good for us. Saturated fat, found in animal fat, coconut and palm oil, is associated with an increased risk of heart disease and certain forms of cancer. A diet high in fat is also associated with obesity because of the high contribution it makes to our overall calorie intake.

Some foods are easily recognised as being high in fat. These include foods such as butter, oil, fried food, fat on meat, roast potatoes, crisps, fried fish, chips and other foods which have been fried. Some foods however, contain 'hidden' fat, such as cakes and biscuits, nuts, full-fat milk, cheese and ice-cream. The principal sources of fat in our diet are meat and meat products (24 per cent); cereal products including biscuits, cakes, pastries, puddings and ice-cream (19 per cent); milk and cheese (15 per cent) and fat spreads (16 per cent).

Fat found in food is termed *saturated, monounsaturated* or *polyunsaturated* depending on its chemical composition. Regardless of whether it is saturated or unsaturated, fat is much higher in calories than either protein or carbohydrate – there are 9 kcalories (kcal) in every gram of fat compared to 4 kcal per gram of protein or 3.75 kcal per gram of carbohydrate.

Fatty acids are the basic units from which fat is made up. There is a perception that all fat is bad for you because fat is high in calories and can cause heart disease. However, two fatty acids which the body cannot make and must be obtained from food are essential. These two 'essential' polyunsaturated fatty acids are called *linoleic acid* and *alpha-linolenic acid*. The British Nutrition Foundation Task Force (1992) and the World Health Organisation have recommended that women planning pregnancy, and those already pregnant, should have an adequate intake of the essential fatty acids. The optimum amount of essential fatty acids required for pregnancy is not known but it is thought that most people living in Britain will be having sufficient to satisfy their needs. Foods which contain these are generally of vegetable origin and include vegetable oils, such as sunflower and corn oil, green leafy vegetables, nuts and seeds. Lean meat, eggs and oily fish, such as mackerel, herrings and salmon, also contain beneficial derivatives of these essential fatty acids.

The general advice about fat in relation to healthy eating is, reduce your saturated fat intake and, if your weight is appropriate for your height (see Appendix 2), replace those calories obtained from fat with more starchy and high fibre foods, such as wholegrain bread, pasta and rice, and vegetables, such as potatoes, carrots and pulses.

Carbohydrate

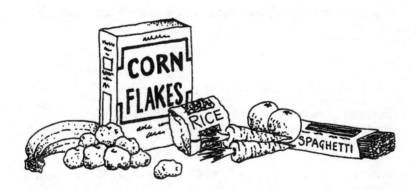

Throughout this century, the proportion of our diet that comes from carbohydrate has lessened considerably and those calories have been replaced by fat. This imbalance has been compounded by the simultaneous change in the type of carbohydrate we eat. At the turn of the century, most of the carbohydrate in the British diet came from 'complex' carbohydrate, in foods such as potatoes, bread and beans – foods which are naturally good sources of vitamins and minerals, particularly if you choose the wholegrain versions of cereal foods. Today, a major proportion of our carbohydrate comes from refined and processed sugars.

Broadly speaking, carbohydrates are made up from starches, sugars and fibre. Although the requirement for carbohydrate is not affected by pregnancy, the message relating to healthy eating in general is that we should eat more unrefined or 'complex' carbohydrate, which means more starchy and high-fibre foods. We should also have less sugar and high-sugar foods. This greater emphasis on starchy foods, fruit and vegetables is central to healthy eating.

Foods which contain a lot of sugar (e.g. jams, confectionery, fizzy drinks) tend to be foods which have been highly processed and are low in vitamins and minerals. They also tend to be foods which contain substantial amounts of fat, especially saturated fat (e.g. biscuits, cakes, pastries, chocolate) and so are high in calories but low in nutrients.

The table below shows that wholegrain cereals have at least double the fibre, vitamin and mineral content of their refined equivalents, for the same number of calories.

NUTRIENT DENSITY PER 250 KCAL OF WHOLE AND REFINED STARCHY FOODS

	Bread		Rice boiled		Pasta boiled	
	wholemeal	white	brown	white	wholemeal	white
Fibre (g)	6.7	1.6	1.4	0.2	7.7	2.9
Vitamin B1 (mg)	0.4	0.2	0.3	trace	0.5	trace
Vitamin B3 (mg)	4.8	1.8	2.3	1.6	2.9	1.2
Vitamin B6 (mg)	0.2	0.1	n/a	0.1	0.2	0.1
Iron (mg)	3.1	1.7	0.9	0.4	3.1	1.2
Zinc (mg)	2.1	0.7	1.2	1.2	2.4	1.2
Magnesium (mg)	88	22	76	20	93	36

Data/information from The Composition of Foods, 5th ed. (1991) is reproduced with the permission of the Royal Society of Chemistry and the Controller of Her Majesty's Stationery Office

Fattening potatoes?

Twenty years ago dietitians were advising patients to cut down on carbohydrate foods when trying to cut down on calories. This legacy had led to some confusion about how 'fattening' bread and potatoes are.

In reality, bread, potatoes and other starchy foods such as rice, pasta and yams are relatively low in calories, especially considering the bulk they contribute to our diet. The pitfall is in how much butter, cream, oil or other fat we add to them in cooking. Here are two examples*:

Bread

1 medium slice	= 75 kcal
1 medium slice + average spread butter	= 185 kcal

Potatoes

6 oz boiled new potatoes	= 130 kcal
6 oz roast potatoes	= 250 kcal
6 oz fine-cut chips	= 620 kcal

* Data/information from The Composition of Foods, 5th ed. (1991) is reproduced with the permission of the Royal Society of Chemistry and the Controller of Her Majesty's Stationery Office

Vitamins

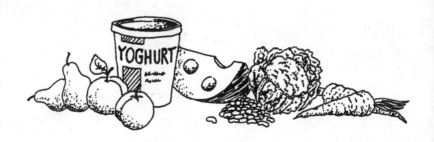

Throughout history, vitamin deficiencies have been a major cause of death and disease. The importance of dietary factors as a cause of disease was not widely recognised until the eighteenth century and it was not until this century that the chemical composition of vitamins was identified.

During the 1930s, the commercial extraction and synthesis of vitamins had begun. The use of vitamins then became fashionable, and sensational claims were made for their curative properties in all types of ailments, many of which went on to be discredited. More recently, government publications and editorials in medical journals, to some extent as a counter to those claims, have played down the value of vitamin supplementation. An exception to the general rule is folic acid at the time of conception, the use of which has provided a dramatic breakthrough in reducing neural tube defects as described earlier in this chapter. The situation is changing again as more sophisticated techniques demonstrate vitamin deficiencies in minority groups of people, even in the most affluent societies.

Vitamins are organic, i.e. they are living compounds and are derived from living material – from plants and animals. They help to regulate the chemical processes that occur in the body and are required in tiny amounts – usually microgram or milligram quantities. The consequence of being organic is that they are easily destroyed and need careful handling when cooking, storing and during food processing.

There are 13 vitamins, each with its own special role to play. These are divided into two groups, the water-soluble and fat-soluble vitamins.

Fat-soluble vitamins	Water-soluble vitamins
	B vitamins
Vitamin A	Thiamin (B1)
Vitamin D	Riboflavin (B2)
Vitamin E	Niacin (B3)
Vitamin K	Pyridoxine (B6)
	Cyanocobolamin (B12)
	Folic acid
	Biotin
	Pantothenic acid
	Vitamin C

Fat-soluble vitamins are stored in the body, so it is not necessary to eat them on a daily basis unless you are eating very small amounts, as may be the case if you are anorexic or on a low-calorie diet. Since these vitamins are stored in the body, they can build up to toxic levels if too much is eaten, hence the cautionary advice on vitamin A and liver for those who are planning pregnancy or who are already pregnant

The water-soluble vitamins, in contrast to the fat-soluble vitamins, are not stored in the body. It is therefore very important to replenish them on a regular basis in a diet containing sufficient foods where these vitamins are found, such as fruit, vegetables, cereals and dairy foods.

Vitamin deficiency

Outward signs of vitamin deficiency are not very common in countries such as Britain but it is important to understand that clinical signs of vitamin deficiencies are the end result of a chain of reactions. In the intervening stages there can be a prolonged period of gradually declining health. For example, the skin and tongue are particularly sensitive to deficiency of B vitamins. If you can observe skin degenerating, it is reasonable to assume that tissue beneath the skin may also have deteriorated.

B vitamins

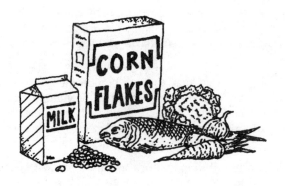

Advertisements for B vitamins might make you believe that they alone will give you energy. This is not true. It is true however, that without B vitamins you may feel tired, because the B vitamins are needed to release energy from the energy yielding nutrients in our food – protein, fat and carbohydrate.

Although each B vitamin has a specific function, it is often difficult to tell which has what effect because the function of one depends on the presence of another. For example, vitamin B12 and folic acid are interdependent, each assisting the other, and deficiency of either causes deficiency signs of both. Similar interdependencies are found between folic acid and thiamin and between riboflavin and a number of B vitamins. For this reason, deficiencies of single B vitamins seldom occur in isolation from other deficiencies, and the wider our choice of foods, the less chance there is of there being a low intake of any essential nutrient.

Pregnancy and B vitamins

The B vitamins, in helping with energy conversion, have a major part to play in new cell formation. They are extremely important at the time of rapid cell division during the first few weeks of pregnancy.

In a study carried out in the East End of London, the maternal intake of B vitamins in the very early part of pregnancy proved to be a strong predictor of birthweight. Low intakes, especially of thiamin and niacin, were associated with lower birthweights – as the mothers ate less, so the size of their babies was smaller. In that study, mothers who had a low intake of thiamin had a ninefold higher probability of having a low-birthweight baby compared to the mothers who had high intakes. The same picture emerged with several other B vitamins including riboflavin and vitamin B6 (Doyle et al., 1990).

The study also showed that above a certain intake, the weight of babies did not go on increasing with higher vitamin intakes. The intakes of mothers with larger babies had, in effect, reached a plateau of 'saturation' which was roughly equal to the Department of Health's recommended intake.

Foods high in the B vitamins are already part of the advice for healthy eating for the general population and include vegetables, wholegrain cereals, lean meat, fish, eggs and milk. The B vitamins are water soluble and are not removed from milk which has a reduced level of fat, i.e. skimmed or semi-skimmed. They are, however, unstable when exposed to heat and to soaking in water.

Folic acid

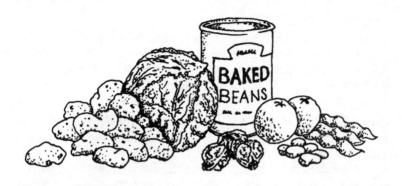

The name 'folic acid' comes from the Latin *folia* (leaf) because it was first found in spinach.

Folic acid plays a fundamental role in cell division, so has obvious implications in situations where rapid cell division is taking place, such as in very early pregnancy. If it is lacking, cell division cannot proceed normally.

Folic acid and the prevention of neural tube defects

The Department of Health recommends that 'women who are planning or who may become pregnant should have a daily 400 mcg folic acid supplement for at least 3 months before conceiving and continue taking it for the first 3 months of pregnancy' (DoH, 1992). They should also eat plenty of folic-acid-rich foods, including foods that have been fortified with folic acid, such as breads and breakfast cereals from which they should expect to obtain another 200 mcg of folic acid a day. This will ensure achieving the recommended daily intake of 600 mcg. If this advice is followed, mothers-to-be will substantially reduce the risk of having a child with a neural tube defect such as *spina bifida* (Wald et al., 1991), as well as other non-genetic abnormalities (Ceizal, 1993).

The mechanism by which folic acid operates is not fully understood but supplementation provided a very high rate of protection in the Medical Research Council study (Wald et al., 1991). Not all neural tube defects (NTD) can be prevented by folic acid supplementation – genetics also plays a part. If either parent has spina bifida, their risk of having a NTD baby is increased tenfold (DoH, 1992). If there is a known case of a neural tube defect, most commonly spina bifida or anencephaly, in either family, it is important to discuss this with your doctor before pregnancy.

Mothers who have had a baby with a neural tube defect have a high risk of a repetition and their doctor will prescribe 5000 mcg of folic acid a day. As *anticonvulsive* drug therapy may be adversely affected by high doses of folic acid, women who suffer from epilepsy must discuss their condition with their doctor.

Only 5 per cent of babies born with a neural tube defect are born to mothers who have had a previous NTD child. This means that most (95 per cent) NTDs are born either to first time mothers or to mothers who have had a previously healthy baby so we have no real clues as to those women who are likely to have a baby suffering from a NTD. For this reason, the Government has recommended a supplement for *all those who wish to become pregnant or who are at risk of becoming pregnant.*

Folic acid supplements (400 mcg) are available from chemists without prescription and cost about £2.50 for two months' supply. Even if you have not had a folic acid supplement before conceiving, start taking one as soon as you realise you are pregnant. The supplement should be taken until the twelfth week of your pregnancy, by which time your baby's neural tube has passed the vulnerable period.

Sources of folic acid

The foods which contain folic acid are the same foods that are always recommended as part of a healthy, well-balanced diet. They include vegetables, particularly green leafy vegetables, potatoes and pulses like baked beans, chick peas, black-eyed beans and lentils; fruit such as citrus fruits, bananas, avocado; bread and cereals, especially wholegrain. Some breads and breakfast cereals are fortified with folic acid, so check the labels. Folic acid is destroyed by heat, so try not to overcook vegetables. It is very unlikely that anyone could ensure a daily intake of 600 mcg folic acid from food sources and it is important to err on the side of caution and take the supplement as well as eating folic-acid-rich foods when planning to become pregnant.

A selected menu providing 600 mcg of folic acid	mcg
Fortified breakfast cereal, 40 g	107
Milk, $\frac{1}{2}$ pint	17
Banana, 1 medium	15
Orange juice, 1 glass	60
Bread, granary, 2 slices	60
Peanut butter, 1 tbs	13
1 pot of yogurt	24
Carrot, raw, 1 medium	25
Chicken, roast, average helping	13
Brussels sprouts, average helping	120
Broccoli, average helping	70
Potato, boiled, average helping	50
Orange, 1	60
	634

Data/information from The Composition of Foods, 5th ed. (1991) is reproduced with the permission of the Royal Society of Chemistry and the Controller of Her Majesty's Stationery Office

Thiamin (vitamin B1)

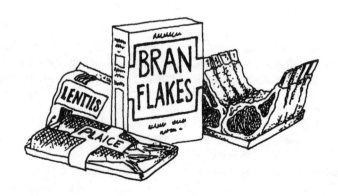

Thiamin is another vitamin which shows a relationship between diet and pregnancy. It was first discovered and isolated in 1937. Prolonged thiamin deficiency results in beriberi and was first observed in the Far East when polished rice became popular. Rice husks, the outer part of the grain, are a rich source of many B vitamins, including thiamin, but when these outer coats of the grain were removed to make the rice whiter and more appealing, beriberi became widespread. A diet severely deficient in thiamin during pregnancy may not adversely affect the mother, but the infant has an increased chance of having beriberi (Van Gelder and Darby, 1944).

Thiamin requirements

The requirement for thiamin is directly related to calorie intake and people who get a lot of their calories from 'empty' calories like sugar and alcohol, which contain few vitamins, have a higher requirement of thiamin. The recommended intake of thiamin for non-pregnant women is 0.8 mg per day, an amount which should also be sufficient to cover pregnancy needs until the third trimester when energy requirements increase; the requirement then increases slightly to 0.9 mg. According to the Dietary Survey of British Adults (Gregory et al., 1990) the majority of women in the UK are having sufficient to cover their needs, but there was a minority whose intakes were below that figure.

Thiamin sources

The most important sources of thiamin are cereal products, which supply 37 per cent of our intake, with vegetables providing a further 25 per cent. Thiamin is present in most foods that are perceived as 'nutritious'. For example, wholegrain or enriched breads, most breakfast cereals, pulses (peas, beans and lentils) and green vegetables are all good sources, as are pork and ham; Quorn, a vegetarian meat substitute is a very rich source (36.6 mg per $3\frac{1}{2}$ oz portion). You can achieve a satisfactory intake by including some of the following foods in your diet:

Recommended intake: 0.8 mg/day	thiamin
Cod's roe, 4 oz/112 g	1.5 mg
Roast pork, 3.5 oz/100 g	0.8 mg
Peanuts, plain 2 oz/50 g	0.6 mg
* Breakfast cereal, fortified, 2 oz/50 g	0.5 mg
Brown, granary or wholemeal bread, 4 slices	0.4 mg
Grilled plaice, 4.5 oz/130 g	0.4 mg

* Check nutrition labels for information.
Data/information from The Composition of Foods, 5th ed. (1991) is reproduced with the permission of the Royal Society of Chemistry and the Controller of Her Majesty's Stationery Office

Riboflavin (vitamin B2)

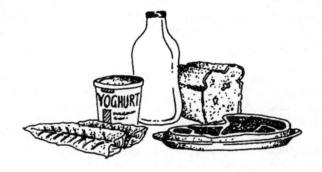

Riboflavin was first described in the 1930s and, like thiamin, helps release energy in every cell of the body. There is no particular disease associated with deficiency of riboflavin but early warning symptoms include cracks around the corners of the mouth and eyes, sensitive inflamed eyelids and painful inflammation of the tongue.

Riboflavin requirements

The recommended daily intake for women is 1.1 mg, with an increase to 1.4 mg during pregnancy. The average intake in the UK is 1.57 mg/day but again, like thiamin, the intakes of some women are much lower than the recommendation. Women who are on a slimming diet have significantly lower levels of riboflavin in their blood than women who are not slimming – another good reason for not restricting dietary intakes when planning to become pregnant.

Riboflavin sources

Milk and milk products are the most valuable source of riboflavin, contributing about 30 per cent of the average UK intake. One pint of milk will provide almost all the riboflavin you need in a day. Riboflavin is easily destroyed by ultra-violet light and much of the riboflavin is lost from bottled milk that is left on the doorstep all day, (especially in the sunshine). Cereal products (22 per cent) and meat and meat products (21 per cent) are also important sources. You can be sure you are getting enough riboflavin by including some of the following foods in your daily diet:

Recommended intake: 1.1 mg/day	riboflavin
Lamb's kidney, fried 3.5 oz/100 g	2.3 mg
* Breakfast cereal, fortified, 2 oz/50 g	0.7 mg
Smoked mackerel, 4 oz/112 g	0.6 mg
Milk, $\frac{1}{2}$ pint	0.5 mg
Yogurt, 1 pot	0.4 mg
Grilled steak, 4 oz/112 g	0.4 mg
Pilchards in tomato sauce, (2)	0.3 mg

* Check nutrition labels for information
Data/information from The Composition of Foods, 5th ed. (1991) is reproduced with the permission of the Royal Society of Chemistry and the Controller of Her Majesty's Stationery Office

Niacin (vitamin B3)

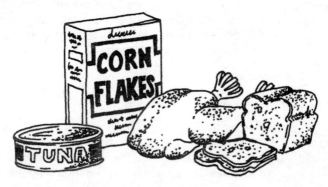

Niacin participates with thiamin and riboflavin in releasing energy from food. It is essential for normal growth and for healthy skin. Niacin deficiency leads to a disease called pellagra, symptoms of which are the three Ds – dermatitis, diarrhoea and dementia. Pellagra became widespread in the Southern States of North America among those who had to subsist on a staple diet of corn, in the early part of this century.

Niacin requirements

Niacin requirements, like thiamin and riboflavin, are related to energy intake. Niacin is unique among the B vitamins in that the body is able to convert tryptophan, a protein, into niacin, as well as obtain it, preformed, from the diet. To make 1 mg of niacin requires approximately 60 mg of tryptophan. Requirements are therefore stated as 'niacin equivalents'. The recommended nutrient intake for niacin is 13 mg a day for women who are not pregnant, an amount also considered to be sufficient to meet the needs of those who are pregnant. The average daily intake in the UK of niacin equivalents is 30 mg for women.

Niacin sources

Niacin is widely distributed in the diet, but found in relatively small amounts. A third of our niacin comes from meat and meat products. Other good sources include wholegrain and enriched bread and breakfast cereals, fish, pulses and nuts. Achieving an adequate intake can be ensured by including some of the following:

Recommended intake: 13 mg/day	niacin
Smoked mackerel, 5 oz/142 g	13.8 mg
Tuna, tinned, 3 oz/85 g	13.6 mg
Brown, granary or wholemeal bread, 4 slices	12.6 mg
Roast chicken or turkey, 4.5 oz/130 g	10.7 mg
Fried lamb's kidney, 3.5 oz/100 mg	9.6 mg
* Breakfast cereal, fortified, 2 oz/50 g	7.5 mg
Peanuts, roast or plain, 50 g packet	6.8 mg

* Check nutrition labels for information.
As you can see, many of the sources are the same as for riboflavin.
Data/information from The Composition of Foods, 5th ed. (1991) is reproduced with the permission of the Royal Society of Chemistry and the Controller of HMSO

Vitamin B6 (Pyridoxine)

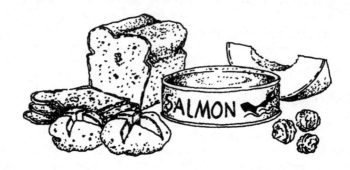

The US Institute of Medicine, in their report on Nutrition during Pregnancy (1990), singled out vitamin B6, along with folic acid, as being the two vitamins most frequently associated with pregnancy complications and adverse outcomes. Vitamin B6 is essential for breaking down ingested protein for use in growth of new body tissues. It is also involved with the production of antibodies and red blood cells. Vitamin B6 supplementation has been found to help some women suffering from premenstrual tension.

Vitamin B6 requirements

Vitamin B6 requirements are related to protein intake, the recommended intake for both pregnant and non-pregnant women is 1.2 mg a day. The average intake of vitamin B6 from food is 1.6 mg a day. There are, however, women whose intakes are below the recommended.

Vitamin B6 sources

Vitamin B6 occurs widely in foods but the best sources are meat, chicken and fish. Other sources include wholegrain and enriched breads and breakfast cereals, potatoes, beans and green vegetables, bananas, melons and peanuts. To achieve the recommended nutrient intake, try to include some of the following foods on a daily basis:

Recommended intake: 1.2 mg/day	vitamin B6
Jacket potato, skin eaten, 6 oz/180 g	0.97 mg
* Breakfast cereal, fortified, 2 oz/50 g	0.90 mg
Steamed salmon, 3.5 oz/100 g	0.83 mg
Tinned tuna, 3.5 oz/100 g	0.50 mg
Stewed rabbit, 3.5 oz/100 g	0.50 mg
Walnuts, 2 oz/50 g	0.33 mg
Banana, 1 medium,	0.30 mg
Avocado pear, ½	0.20 mg

* Check nutrition labels for information.
Data/information from The Composition of Foods, 5th ed. (1991) is reproduced with the permission of the Royal Society of Chemistry and the Controller of Her Majesty's Stationery Office

Vitamin B12 (Cyanocobalomin)

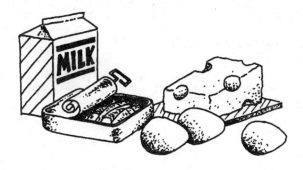

The distinction between B12 and folic acid was unclear until the 1950s. Their roles intertwine but they each serve a specific purpose that the other cannot perform. Vitamin B12 is linked with folic acid in having a central role in the production of red blood cells and the prevention of anaemia. Dietary deficiency of B12 is thought to be relatively rare as it is present in all foods of animal origin, and it is also manufactured by micro-organisms in the intestine. This is the probable source for vegans and vegetarians.

Vitamin B12 requirements

The recommended intake for women is 1.5 mcg per day which is a very tiny amount. The average intake for women in the UK is 5.4 mcg, which suggests that few women are likely to be deficient.

Vitamin B12 sources

Vitamin B12 is unique in being found almost exclusively in foods of animal origin. Anyone who eats meat on a frequent basis is likely to have an adequate intake. Good sources include meat, oily fish such as sardines and pilchards, milk, cheese and eggs. Vegans should seek a reliable source such as meat substitute (e.g. Quorn), a fortified soya milk or a vitamin supplement (see section on vegetarians). A good intake can be assured if some of the following foods are included in the diet on a regular basis:

Recommended intake: 1.5 mcg/day	vitamin B12
Fried lamb's kidney, 3.5 oz/100 g	79.0 mcg
Tinned sardines, 3.5 oz/100 g	28.0 mcg
Stewed rabbit, 3.5 oz/100 g	12.0 mcg
Milk, $\frac{1}{2}$ pint	1.1 mcg
Egg, 1	0.6 mcg
Cheese, most types, 1 oz/25 g	0.3 mcg

Data/information from The Composition of Foods, 5th ed. (1991) is reproduced with the permission of the Royal Society of Chemistry and the Controller of Her Majesty's Stationery Office

Vitamin C

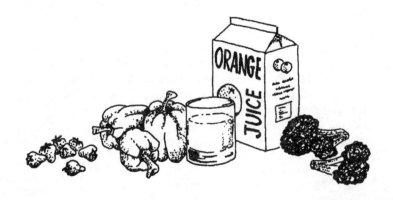

In 1774, a British physician, Dr James Lind, discovered that if sailors with scurvy were given rations of oranges and lemons, they were soon cured and it took another 50 years before all sea-going vessels were required to carry sufficient lime juice for every sailor to receive some daily – hence British sailors were nick-named 'limeys'. Almost two hundred years after Lind's discovery, the 'antiscorbutic' factor was identified and named ascorbic acid or vitamin C.

Vitamin C has numerous functions. It is an important anti-oxidant (protective) vitamin, exerting a protective role in the body's defence mechanism and it helps to maintain the integrity of blood vessels. The early signs of deficiency include gums bleeding easily and small blood vessels under the skin breaking spontaneously, causing tiny haemorrhages.

In pregnancy, vitamin C enhances iron absorption from plant sources by two- to fourfold. Vitamin C deficiency impairs the production of collagen, a protein that gives structure to bones, cartilage, muscle and blood vessels. Vitamin C levels in fetal blood may be 50 per cent higher than in maternal blood as a result of the ability of the placenta to concentrate some nutrients to the benefit of the fetus.

Vitamin C requirements

The recommended intake for women is 40 mg a day, increasing to 50 mg during pregnancy and to 70 mg when breast-feeding. The average intake of women in the UK is 62 mg, although the average intakes of younger women, aged 16 to 24, is markedly lower than that.

Vitamin C sources

The main sources of Vitamin C are from vegetables (46 per cent), drinks, including fruit juices (22 per cent) and fruit (17 per cent). A good supply of vitamin C can be ensured by including some of the following foods on a daily basis:

Recommended intake: 40 mg/day	vitamin C
Fruit	
Stewed blackcurrants, 4 oz/112 g	129 mg
Guava fruit, 2 oz/50 g	115 mg
Strawberries, 4 oz/112 g	86 mg
Orange, medium size	86 mg
Orange juice, $\frac{1}{4}$ pint	55 mg
Kiwi fruit, medium size	35 mg
Vegetables	
Pepper, raw, half	96 mg
Spring greens, 3·5 oz/100 g	77 mg
Brussels sprouts, 3·5 oz/100 g	60 mg
Broccoli, 3·5 oz/100 g	44 mg
New potatoes, boiled in skins, 6 oz/180 g	27 mg
Old potatoes, boiled in skins, 6 oz/180 g	11 mg

Data/information from The Composition of Foods, 5th ed. (1991) is reproduced with the permission of the Royal Society of Chemistry and the Controller of Her Majesty's Stationery Office

Vitamin C is easily destroyed by heat, by leaching into water during cooking and by exposure to oxygen in the air. Vegetables that are to be cooked should therefore not be chopped more than necessary or left to soak in water. They should be cooked in small amounts of water or steamed for as short a time as possible. Much of the vitamin C is stored just under the skin of vegetables, so more will be preserved if, for instance, potatoes are left unpeeled.

Fat-soluble vitamins

Vitamin A

Although uncommon in the UK, vitamin A deficiency results in up to 500,000 cases of blindness or impaired vision every year, primarily in children in the Third World. Along with iodine deficiency, this provides another example where a cheap remedy is available to cure a condition for which the cause is established, but the political will is lacking.

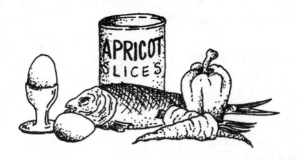

Besides its role in the visual system, vitamin A is also an essential component in promoting cell growth and appears to be important in fetal growth. A low maternal blood level of vitamin A is associated with premature birth, growth retardation and low birthweight.

Vitamin A requirements

The recommended intake for women is 600 mcg a day which is not difficult to achieve – the average intake for women in the UK is 1490 mcg a day.

Vitamin A sources

Vitamin A is found in animal foods as retinol (preformed vitamin A) and in plant foods as beta-carotene which the body can convert to vitamin A. It takes 6 mcg of beta-carotene to make 1 mcg of retinol.

Retinol is found in very high concentrations in liver (see 'Caution' below). It is also found in fatty fish such as herring and mackerel, and in egg yolk, full-fat milk, butter, cheese and margarines which, by law, have to be fortified with vitamins A and D.

Carotene is found in yellow, red and leafy dark-green vegetables such as carrots, red peppers, spinach and spring greens; it is also found in yellow and red fruits such as apricots, mangoes, cantaloupe melons and sharon fruit.

Recommended intake: 600 mcg/day	vitamin A
	retinol equivalents
Animal sources (retinol)	
Fried lambs' kidney, 3.5 oz/100 g	110
Boiled egg	95
Cheese, full-fat types, 1 oz/25 g	81
Kipper, 4.5 oz/130 g	43
Plant sources (beta-carotene)	
Carrots, 3.5 oz/100 g	1260
Sweet potato, 3.5 oz/100 g	660
Spinach, 3 oz/100 g	640
Red pepper, $\frac{1}{2}$	576
Mango, 3.5 oz/100 g	300
Melon, cantaloupe, 3.5 oz/100 g	167

Data/information from The Composition of Foods, 5th ed. (1991) is reproduced with the permission of the Royal Society of Chemistry and the Controller of Her Majesty's Stationery Office

CAUTION!

Women trying to conceive are advised by the Department of Health not to take supplements and/or fish oil capsules containing vitamin A, unless advised by their doctor. Vitamin supplements prescribed as part of antenatal care contain safe levels of vitamin A (400 to 1250 mcg) and can be taken safely.

Vitamin A deficiency is detrimental to your unborn child but large doses of vitamin A, particularly early in pregnancy, can also be harmful. There is evidence suggesting that a vitamin A intake in excess of 8000 to 10,000 mcg a day may cause birth defects, however, only one such case has been reported. This was the case of an American woman who had an abnormally high intake of vitamin A. Taken overall, the risk of birth defects from an excess dietary intake is very low; birth defects must be viewed as the extreme consequences. For peace of mind, it is best to err on the side of caution and follow the advice of the Department of Health.

There is a risk of excessive intakes of vitamin A from liver. In recent years, the vitamin A content of animal liver has increased considerably, probably due to changes in feeding practices. A 100 g (3½ oz) portion of liver contains between 20,000 and 40,000 mcg, depending on the animal. This is unacceptably high when you consider the upper safe level (8000 to 10,000 mcg/day) set in relation to prevention of birth defects. The Department of Health has therefore also recommended that **women who are trying to become pregnant or who are pregnant should avoid eating liver and liver products such as pâté and liver sausage.**

Other food sources of vitamin A (e.g. margarine, dairy produce and eggs or yellow vegetables) do not pose any risk from excessive intakes.

Vitamin D

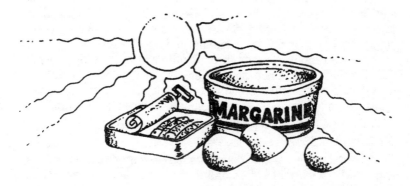

Vitamin D is necessary for normal growth and for the growth and maintenance of bones and teeth. It also helps in the absorption of calcium.

Vitamin D sources

Vitamin D is produced in the body by the action of sunlight on the skin. Even in the UK, most people exposed to the sun are capable of satisfying their requirements for the summer and building up enough reserves, stored in the liver, to last through the winter months. For those who do not spend time outside, such as the housebound, it will be necessary to obtain their vitamin D from dietary sources. These include fatty fish such as pilchards and sardines, eggs and margarines.

Vitamin D requirements

Because sufficient vitamin D is obtained by adults from sunshine, no recommended intake has been set for dietary sources of vitamin D. However, lower levels of vitamin D are found on the fetal side of the placenta than the maternal side. To avoid low levels in your baby, it is recommended that you should have a minimum of 10 mcg of vitamin D daily. A supplement may be required to achieve that amount, particularly if your fat intake is low.

Minerals

Minerals, unlike vitamins, are inorganic elements. They are stable and are unaffected by heat; they 'exist' elementally or forever. When you cook a food that contains vitamins and minerals, the compounds that make up vitamins undergo restructuring, often causing the vitamins to lose their identity and be destroyed, while the minerals remain unchanged. Minerals can, however, be difficult to absorb into the body from food, but absorption is often helped by ensuring you have an adequate supply of specific vitamins; for example vitamin C helps iron absorption and vitamin D helps calcium absorption.

The minerals which will be discussed here are those that have been found to be important before and during pregnancy. They include magnesium, calcium, iron and zinc. Other minerals are not included for discussion because there is very little likelihood of anyone in the UK being deficient in them as normal intakes in the UK are well above the recommended intake, or because they have not been found to be especially important in relation to pregnancy. These minerals include sodium, chloride, potassium, phosphorus, copper, iodine, selenium, manganese, fluoride, chromium, molybdenum, arsenic, nickel, silicon and boron.

Magnesium

Magnesium, along with calcium, is present in both the body and our diet in much larger amounts than other trace elements such as iron.

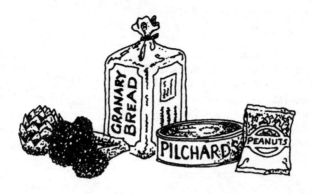

Magnesium is an essential component of all the cells of soft tissues, where it forms part of the protein-building mechanism. It is also essential for the release of energy. It was the mineral most closely associated with birthweight in the East London study (Doyle et al., 1990) which found that premature birth and the risk of low birthweight was increased with low intakes of magnesium early in pregnancy. A follow-up study concluded that supplementation with magnesium after 13 weeks of pregnancy failed to have a significant effect on birthweight (Doyle et al., 1992). This suggests that an adequate intake of magnesium may be more important around the time of conception when rapid cell division is taking place, than in the second or third trimesters.

Magnesium requirements

The recommended intake for magnesium is 270 mg a day for women; the average intake of magnesium is 237 mg. It is therefore thought that an important minority of women in the UK would benefit from a higher intake, especially around the time of conception.

Magnesium sources

Magnesium is widely distributed in foods, especially wholegrain cereals, dark green vegetables, pulses, nuts, seeds and in seafood. More than 80 per cent of magnesium in cereals is found in the germ and outer layers of the grain. Unrefined cereals are therefore a much richer source of magnesium. Adequate supplies of magnesium will be achieved by including in your diet some of the following foods on a regular basis:

Recommended intake: 270 mg/day	magnesium
Sunflower seeds, 2 tbs	139 mg
Peanuts, plain or roast, 2 oz/50 g	90 mg
Brown, granary or wholemeal bread, 4 slices	83 mg
* Breakfast cereal, fortified, 40 g	65 mg
Pilchards, tinned 3.5 oz/100 g	39 mg
Boiled lentils, 3.5 oz/100 g	34 mg
Spinach, 3·5 oz/100 g	34 mg

* Check nutrition labels for information.
Data/information from The Composition of Foods, 5th ed. (1991) is reproduced with the permission of the Royal Society of Chemistry and the Controller of Her Majesty's Stationery Office

Calcium

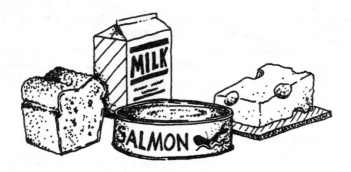

Calcium is the most abundant mineral in the body, 99 per cent of which is found in the bones.

There is no evidence that calcium requirements are increased during pregnancy, but low calcium intakes threaten the integrity of maternal bones. There is a concern about the possible effects of low intakes of pregnant women, particularly in those under the age of 25, in whom bone mineralisation (hardening) may still be taking place. Because bone density appears to diminish in the first three months of pregnancy (Purdie, 1989), it seems sensible for all women to build up a calcium reserve in advance of pregnancy. Calcium concentrations are higher in the developing fetus than in the mother (Reeve, 1991) which suggests that your baby will maintain an adequate supply at your expense!

Calcium requirements

The recommended calcium intake for women is 700 mg a day. The average intake of women in the UK, aged 16 to 34, is 689 mg; this means that a substantial number of women have intakes less than that recommended.

Calcium sources

Almost half our calcium is obtained from milk and cheese and a quarter comes from bread and other cereals. One pint of milk a day will almost supply the recommended intake. Other sources include yogurt, tinned fish such as sardines, where the bones are eaten, dark-green vegetables, bread and figs.

Recommended intake : 700 mg/day	calcium
Whitebait, 3.5 oz/100 g	860 mg
Milk, full- or low-fat, 1 pint	680 mg
Sardines, tinned, 4 sardines, 3.5 oz/100 g	550 mg
Tofu (soya bean curd) steamed, 3.5 oz/100 g	510 mg
Pilchards, 2, 3.5 oz/100 g	300 mg
Cheese, hard types, 1 oz/25 g	210 mg
Spinach, 3.5 oz/100 g	160 mg

Data/information from The Composition of Foods, 5th ed. (1991) is reproduced with the permission of the Royal Society of Chemistry and the Controller of Her Majesty's Stationery Office

Iron

Iron is vital for cell respiration – the process by which cells generate energy. It is also needed in making new cells and hormones and forms a large part of haemoglobin, the oxygen-carrying protein in red blood cells.

Menstrual losses make a woman's iron needs much greater than the needs of a man. About 40 per cent of women aged 18 to 34 have low blood iron stores. Even if a woman has not been diagnosed as iron deficient, she is likely to be prone to deficiency and should therefore pay special attention to her diet in an effort to

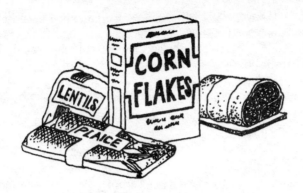

maintain her iron stores. Iron deficiency, the cause of which is usually poor nutrition, can be very debilitating, leading to apathy, tiredness and poor tolerance to cold.

During pregnancy, the placenta can deliver large quantities of iron to the baby, even if it means depriving you of iron. Anaemic women have a greater chance of premature delivery and increased infant mortality (Kitay and Habort, 1975).

Iron requirements

The recommended iron intake for women is 14.8 mg a day. The average intake among women in the UK is 10.5 mg per day, so there are many women who are not reaching the target. Requirements are not increased during pregnancy because there is no loss of iron through menstruation, and absorption of iron is enhanced during pregnancy.

Iron absorption

To obtain sufficient iron from food, it is necessary not only to choose foods that are rich in iron but also to select foods rich in vitamin C which helps absorption.

Sources of iron

There are two sources of iron in the diet – *'heme'* iron, from animal protein, and *'non-heme'* iron from plant sources. The best sources of absorbable heme iron come from meat, particularly offal such as heart, kidney and oxtail (remember, liver, although a rich source of iron and many other nutrients, is not recommended because of the high vitamin A content). Lean meat, chicken and fish all contain moderate amounts while milk and cheese contain very little. The iron in eggs is poorly absorbed.

Plant sources of iron (non-heme) include cereals – enriched breakfast cereals, wholegrain bread and cereals and vegetables – dark-green vegetables such as spring greens; despite Popeye's faith in spinach, the iron in it is not well absorbed.

Recommended intake: 14.8 mg/day	iron
Black pudding, 3 oz/100 g	20.0 mg
Fried lamb's kidney, 3.5 oz/100 g	12.0 mg
Grilled lean steak, 8 oz/225 g	7.7 mg
Boiled lentils, 3 tbs	4.2 mg
* Breakfast cereal, fortified, 2 oz/50 g	3.3 mg
Red kidney beans, 3 tbs	2.1 mg
Spinach, 3.5 oz/100 g	1.6 mg

* Check nutrition labels for information – some contain more.
Data/information from The Composition of Foods, 5th ed. (1991) is reproduced with the permission of the Royal Society of Chemistry and the Controller of Her Majesty's Stationery Office

Zinc

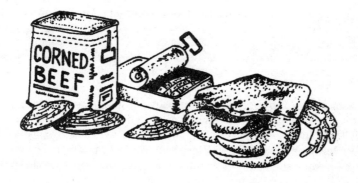

Zinc is involved in the process of cell replication and differentiation, and it is therefore important to have a good supply in the early stages of pregnancy.

An adequate reserve of maternal zinc is essential for normal embryonic and fetal development in animals (Hurley and Mutch, 1973), with low intakes being associated with higher rates of miscarriage. A number of studies have found that women with low serum zinc levels had an increased incidence of babies with congenital malformations of the central nervous system (Wharton, 1992). Low intakes early in pregnancy have also been related to growth retardation and lower birthweights (Jameson, 1976).

Zinc also seems to be important for the father since zinc is an important component of sperm and increases sperm mobility, adding to the chance of conception. Zinc deficiency is common in Iran, Egypt and elsewhere in the Middle East where the diet is usually low in animal products.

Zinc sources

Foods rich in zinc are also good sources of other nutrients. The main sources of zinc in our diet are high-protein foods of animal origin and, like iron, zinc from vegetables is less well absorbed. Zinc competes with iron for absorption and its absorption can therefore be compromised by iron supplementation. Long-term use of oral contraceptives may also reduce plasma zinc levels, although evidence of this is slight.

Those most likely to be at risk of zinc deficiency are vegetarians and vegans, long-term users of oral contraception and those who participate in strenuous exercise (zinc is lost through sweat glands).

Zinc requirements

Extra zinc is required during pregnancy, but because of increased absorption of zinc, it is thought that healthy women adapt metabolically to ensure that an adequate amount of zinc is transferred to the developing baby. The dietary requirement for zinc in pregnancy is therefore the same as for non-pregnant women, that is 7 mg a day.

Recommended intake: 7 mg/day	zinc
Oysters, half dozen	27.0 mg
Stewed beef, 3.5 oz/100 g	8.7 mg
Roast lamb, 3.5 oz/100 g	5.3 mg
Corned beef, 3.5 oz/100 g	5.6 mg
Crab, 3.5 oz/100 g	5.5 mg
Sardines, 4	3.0 mg

Data/information from The Composition of Foods, 5th ed. (1991) is reproduced with the permission of the Royal Society of Chemistry and the Controller of Her Majesty's Stationery Office

Supplements

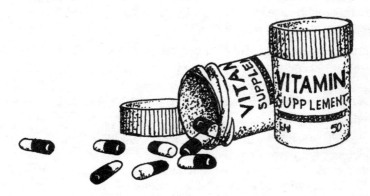

Many people are, understandably, unsure that they meet their nutritional needs from food alone. In theory of course, anyone who eats a healthy, well-balanced diet should not need supplements, but how many of us can claim we eat a healthy diet all of the time?

The Department of Health has recommended that all those who are trying to conceive or who could be pregnant should take a daily supplement of 400 mcg of folic acid (see page 27). They have also suggested a supplement of vitamin D during pregnancy to achieve an intake of 10 mcg/day. Any other decisions on whether to take a supplement are left to the individual.

Reasons for taking supplements

The Dietary Survey of British Adults detected a proportion of the population with low intakes of vitamins and minerals. The incidence is low but it provides grounds for arguing that some people may need nutritional supplements. It can further be argued that if symptoms of deficiencies can be detected, then marginal deficiencies which go undetected may affect a much larger number. This group is likely to be 'below par', neither feeling nor functioning well.

Within the child-bearing age-group, marginal deficiencies may arise among:

- habitual dieters with low calorie intakes
- women with heavy periods
- those who may be emotionally or physically unwell and who lose their appetite
- strict vegetarians
- those who eat monotonous or bizarre diets, such as food faddists
- those who have illnesses that impair absorption of nutrients
- those on limited income.

Anyone falling into any of these categories will probably benefit from a wide-ranging vitamin/mineral supplement.

Arguments against taking supplements

The principal argument against taking supplements is that they can create a belief in the user that 'I can eat what I like because my supplement will cover my needs'. Although a prerequisite of a healthy diet is an adequate intake of vitamins and minerals, this is only a part of the story; when taken out of context it can erode the underlying needs for a balanced diet. The amounts of energy, protein, carbohydrate and fat all need to be taken into account when planning a healthy diet.

A second objection is an argument against high or 'mega' doses of supplements, particularly of single nutrients other than that of folic acid, While vitamins and minerals are essential to good health, it does not follow that more of what is good for you is better. High doses of most nutrients pose dangers. Personal tolerance levels of high doses vary in the same way as thresholds for deficiencies vary.

A third problem is absorption of supplements. When vitamins and minerals are absorbed from food, they are present with other components that may help with their absorption. When supplements, particularly minerals, are taken in a large dose and in a concentrated form, they can often interfere with the absorption of other essential nutrients. Notably, zinc interferes with calcium absorption, iron with zinc absorption, calcium with iron and magnesium absorption, and magnesium with the absorption of calcium and iron. Similarly some nutrients can enhance the absorption of others, as in the case of vitamin C and iron and vitamin D and calcium. Therefore taking supplements of one without the other may be ineffectual.

Due to these objections, the nutrient needs of healthy individuals should be met by choosing a variety of foods, rather than by supplementation, thus reducing the potential risk of both excesses and deficiencies.

Choosing a supplement

Having considered the arguments above, you may still feel you want to take a supplement; so how do you decide which to choose? Unless your doctor advises you to the contrary, it is best to look for a single balanced vitamin/mineral supplement, made by a reputable manufacturer or an own-brand supermarket supplement. European Union rulings are making it more difficult for manufacturers to make spurious claims about such things as 'vitality', 'improving sporting achievements' or 'stress reduction'. It is still, however, a little bewildering to look at all the information on the labels and wonder what to choose.

The first question to ask is: what vitamins and minerals do I need? Concentrate on the list of nutrients and the amount of each nutrient as a percentage of the RDA (recommended daily intake).

- Choose a preparation which contains a wide range of the B vitamins and vitamin C, iron, zinc, magnesium. Our requirement for calcium is high in terms of volume (almost 1 gram a day) so it is unlikely that multivitamin/mineral preparations will contain the RDA for calcium.
- Avoid supplements with a high vitamin A content (not more than 1250 mcg per day from supplement).
- Avoid supplements that provide more than 100 per cent of the RDA. Remember, you are eating food as well, so at least part of your needs will be met from food.

- Avoid supplements with high iron concentrations (not more than 10 mg). Iron overload can cause problems just as deficiency can.
- Avoid 'organic' or 'natural' supplements. Your purse will know the difference but your body won't.
- Avoid preparations that contain non-essential nutrients such as inositol and choline. These won't do any harm but suggest a suspect marketing strategy that could also reflect on the product itself.
- Chewable varieties of supplements are more readily absorbed.

There is a serious lack of control on health food products, with an unsuspecting consumer often left uninformed. Preparations of 'mega' amounts of individual nutrients are readily available for the trusting customer to buy, which in most circumstances are of little use and usually expensive.

Examples of what one might consider indefensible doses include vitamin E and vitamin B6: vitamin E is available to be bought over-the-counter in 1000 mg doses when detrimental effects are known to occur in some people consuming 400 mg a day. An optimum intake level has not been set in the UK for vitamin E but the American recommended allowance for adult women is 8 mg a day. To obtain 1000 mg of vitamin E from the richest food source we have, wheatgerm, you would have to eat 10 lb of wheatgerm. Similarly, excessive doses can be bought of most nutrients – 100 mg vitamin B6, recommended intake is 1.2 mg/day; 5000 mg vitamin C, recommended intake 40 mg/day. To obtain 5000 mg of vitamin C from food you would need to eat 29 lb of oranges!

Nature clearly did not expect, or biologically prepare, us to have mega doses of micronutrients. If food can provide us with all the nutrients we need, why not get them from food? Food has so much more to recommend it!

Vegetarian diets

Ecological, humane and health benefits have attracted many people to vegetarianism. If well planned, a vegetarian can have a perfectly healthy diet, achieving all their nutrient requirements.

In the East London study, the consumption of meat was similar in the low-birthweight group of mothers to that of the mothers who had optimum-birthweight babies (Wynn et al., 1991). This suggests that low meat consumption was not a risk factor for this particular population. However, the duration of pregnancy has been found to be four or five days shorter and babies are lighter in Hindu vegetarians than in Muslim or white women (Saunders and Reddy, 1994). Lower birthweights have also been reported in white communities consuming macrobiotic diets and for vegans. It is thought this may be due to low intake of iron or folic acid and vitamin B12.

Vegetarians who regularly eat dairy foods and eggs can obtain energy and all the essential amino acids and other nutrients that they will need for a healthy pregnancy. Vegans, however, who eat no animal products, will need to plan their diet much more carefully if they are not to suffer from deficiencies. Nutrients likely to be low in a vegan diet, and which are especially important for those preparing for or who are already pregnant, include essential amino acids from animal protein foods, calcium, iron, zinc, vitamin B2 and vitamin B12.

It is important to eat **a variety of plant protein foods** including pulses, nuts and seeds and a wide range of cereal grains. In this way, the proteins found in one plant will be complemented with the proteins in other plants.

3

ASSESSING YOUR DIET

'Input'   'Output'

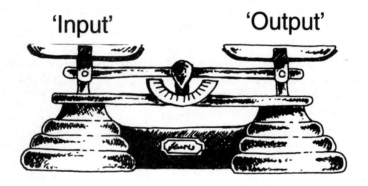

You can use this chapter to assess how your usual food intake and eating habits compare with the recommendations on healthy eating. These recommendations are based upon the daily diets of women who had good-sized healthy babies in a study carried out in London (Wynn et al., 1991) and the current government recommendations (Dietary Reference Values – DRVs). The chapter is divided into two sections, a self-assessment questionnaire and a food diary to fill in what you eat each day, for seven days.

The question and answer assessment takes a fairly general look at your usual eating pattern. It is followed by an answer section which takes on a fictitious character called 'Ms Ideal', who fills in the self-assessment questionnaire. Reasons for why Ms Ideal's usual eating habits are healthy are given.

Diet assessment questionnaire

1 Do you normally eat three meals a day?   **Yes/No**

2 Do you eat breakfast cereals more than three times a week?   **Yes/No**

3 Do you normally drink 1 pint of milk (or more) each day?   **Yes/No**

4 Do you like: yogurt?   **Yes/No**

                              cheese?   **Yes/No**

5 What sort of bread do you usually eat?   **Wholemeal/Brown/White**

6 Do you eat sandwiches?   **Yes/No**

7 How many times a week do you eat lean red meat,

   such as beef, lamb or pork?   ____ **per week**

8 How many units of alcohol do you have in a week?   ____ **units**

   (1 unit = 1 glass of wine, 1 measure of spirits, $\frac{1}{2}$ pint of beer)

9 Are there any foods you do not eat, e.g. milk, meat?   Yes/No

   a) _____ b) _____ c) _____

10 Do you take any vitamin or other supplements   **Yes/No**

11 How often do you eat liver?   ____ **times/month**

12 Do you eat a portion of potatoes/rice/pasta each day?   **Yes/No**

13 How many portions of vegetable (excluding potatoes)

    do you eat each week?   ____

14 How many pieces of fruit do you have each week?   ____

15 How many cups of tea or coffee do you have a day?   ____ **cups**

16 How many teaspoons of sugar do you use in tea/coffee?   ____

17 What type of milk do you drink?   **Whole/semi-skimmed/skimmed**

18 How many times a week do you have fried foods?   ____ **times**

19 How many times a week do you eat sweet or savoury
    snacks (e.g. chocolates, cakes, pastries, biscuits, crisps)?   ____ **times**

The seven day food diary is a more in-depth way of assessing your food intake and requires a little more commitment to complete. It will show whether your diet is likely to meet the recommendations for healthy eating when planning pregnancy.

The main purpose of this assessment is to look at your protein and complex carbohydrate intakes from five different food groups. If you are having enough servings from each of the groups, then the likelihood is that you are having an adequate intake of calories, protein, vitamins and minerals which, after all, is what is most important when planning pregnancy. The exercise will not consider your fat and sugar intakes. Most of us eat too much fat and refined sugar, so cutting down on these should be an integral part of healthy eating for everyone. If your weight is appropriate for your height but you do eat fried and/or high-fat, low-nutrient foods such as crisps, biscuits, pastry, chocolate etc., you may wish to consider cutting down on these and replacing those calories from food in the food groups mentioned below, which will provide you with many more vitamins and minerals. If you are overweight, try to get that under control at least three months before trying to conceive, again by concentrating on reducing the amount of fat and sugar in your diet.

What does the dietary assessment tell you?

Let's assume that a fictitious Ms Ideal, who is planning to have a baby, filled in the questionnaire. She is called Ms Ideal because she is 'perfect' although, as we all know, perfection or the ideal does not exist. Ms Ideal is simply our model mum-of-the-future. You can use her answers to the questionnaire as a guide to the 'ideal' diet; but don't feel guilty if you don't measure up to her!

Q.1 Ms Ideal eats three meals a day It is really quite difficult to get all the vitamins and minerals you need in less than three meals a day. Snacking throughout the day may provide the calories you need, but is unlikely to provide you with enough vitamins and minerals – snack foods are often high in calories and low in vitamins and minerals. If you are underweight it is particularly important that you eat three meals a day plus snacks.

Q.2 Ms Ideal eats breakfast cereals more than three times a week The Hackney study found that women who had breakfast cereals regularly had (a) a higher vitamin and mineral intake because breakfast cereals are usually fortified with B vitamins and some minerals and (b) they had a much higher probability of having a healthy, good-sized baby (Doyle, 1990).

Q.3 Ms Ideal has 1 pint of milk every day Milk is the nearest thing to a perfect food although it is low in iron and high in saturated fat. It contains high-quality protein and is a very good source of calcium, vitamin B2 (riboflavin), vitamin B12 and phosphorus. One pint of milk supplies Ms Ideal with almost all she needs of calcium and riboflavin, more than half her vitamin A and vitamin B12, and more than a third of her protein requirements.

Q.4 Ms Ideal likes both yogurt and cheese They are both good sources of the same nutrients as milk. It would therefore be a good idea to include these as a regular part of your diet. If you did not eat any of these dairy foods you could be at risk of being deficient in calcium, which is important for strong bones and teeth. Q. 10 is important to you.

Q.5 Ms Ideal eats wholemeal bread Brown, and even more so, wholemeal bread, is much higher than white bread in fibre, B vitamins, magnesium, iron and zinc, all of which are important when planning pregnancy.

Q.6 Ms Ideal eats sandwiches most days for her lunch They are quick, easy to prepare and with the right fillings they are very tasty and nutritious.

Q.7 Ms Ideal eats meat 2–3 times a week Red meat is a good source of the kind of iron which our bodies can absorb easily. If you eat meat less frequently or not at all Q. 10 is important to you.

Q.8 Ms Ideal does not drink any alcohol It is a good idea for both you and your partner to reduce alcohol intake during the planning stages of pregnancy. Excessive alcohol can lead to sperm damage and to a low sperm count. The fertilised egg, in the very early stages of pregnancy, is especially vulnerable to damage from maternal alcohol excesses.

Q.9 Ms Ideal eats everything There will of course be good reasons why some people do not eat certain foods; religious beliefs, moral considerations, allergies and other medical conditions are all grounds for dietary restrictions. Not eating from a particular food group makes you more susceptible to deficiencies in essential nutrients. If you do avoid groups of foods such as meat, and do not take care to make good possible deficiencies, you must ensure you get reliable advice about which nutrients you could be lacking in, and which foods are good sources of those nutrients. Q.10 may be important to you.

Q.10 Ms Ideal takes a supplement of folic acid (400 mcg) every day. She also takes a multivitamin and mineral pill occasionally when she feels she has not had time to eat well, i.e. eating foods from each of the five food groups If you feel that you don't always eat a variety of foods, an occasional 'top-up' with a multivitamin and mineral supplement can be a good idea.

The Department of Health recommends that every woman who is planning to become pregnant should start taking a **400 mcg folic acid supplement** three months before conceiving and for the first three months of her pregnancy (DoH, 1992). Folic acid significantly reduces the risk of having a baby born with a neural tube defect such as spina bifida. They also recommend eating foods rich in folic acid, such as fortified breakfast cereals (look at the label), green leafy vegetables and oranges.

If you are a vegetarian or vegan, or you do not eat red meat (source of easily absorbed iron), or dairy foods (a source of calcium) it is a good idea to take a multivitamin and mineral supplement when planning to become pregnant to ensure you have enough of these essential nutrients. If you are taking anything other than folic acid and a multivitamin/mineral supplement, do consult your doctor or a dietitian.

Q.11 Ms Ideal has stopped eating liver Liver contains very high levels of vitamin A which could potentially damage the baby. The government have therefore recommended that women who are pregnant or who are planning to have a baby should avoid eating liver, including liver pâté and liver sausage, during that time.

Q.12 Ms Ideal always has potatoes, rice or pasta each day with her main meal These provide fibre and a variety of water-soluble vitamins. They also provide bulk to her diet. Brown rice or whole-wheat pasta contain more fibre and vitamins than their white counterparts. These nutrients would also be provided by cassava, yams, sweet potatoes, plantains and other root vegetables and tubers.

Q.13 Ms Ideal eats two vegetables or a large salad, as well as potatoes, every day Vegetables provide fibre and are valuable sources of many vitamins and minerals. Green leafy vegetables are especially good as they contain folic acid, vitamin C, carotene, iron, magnesium and other trace elements.

Q.14 Ms Ideal eats, on average, two pieces of fruit each day but sometimes has a glass of fresh orange juice as an alternative Like vegetables, fruit provides fibre as well as valuable vitamins such as vitamin C and varying amounts of the B vitamins. Yellow fruits such as apricots, peaches and mangoes are good sources of carotene. Dried fruits are good sources of iron and other trace elements.

Q.15 Ms Ideal drinks fewer than four cups of tea or coffee a day Although there is no hard evidence against caffeine and pregnancy outcome, recent research has found that women who had excessive amounts of caffeine in their diet had a higher risk of miscarriage.

The remainder of these questions and answers are only important if you are overweight and want to lose weight before your pregnancy. If you are overweight, the best approach to losing it is to cut down on foods that are high in fat and sugar. The following questions are answered as if Ms Ideal has changed her diet in order to lose weight. Remember you should stop dieting at least three months before conceiving.

Q.16 Ms Ideal either uses a sweetener or does not add anything to her tea and coffee Sugar contains calories and not much else. Try to cut back a little each day until you can stop altogether.

Q.17 Ms Ideal has skimmed milk Skimmed milk has virtually no fat but most of the goodness of whole milk, i.e. the calcium, phosphorus, vitamin B2 and protein. In choosing skimmed milk she has halved her calorie intake from milk (186 kcal per pint of skimmed milk).

Q.18 Ms Ideal eats fried foods very occasionally Fried foods contain a lot of fat and therefore can contribute a lot of calories to your diet. Try to grill, bake, boil or steam foods that you are used to frying.

Q.19 Ms Ideal seldom eats sweet or savoury snacks She has three meals a day so does not often feel the need to snack between meals. It is hard to resist your favourite chocolate bar or piece of cake, but try just to allow yourself one or two treats a week, possibly at the weekend. If you do feel hungry between meals, have an orange or other fruit. We often eat out of boredom, so find something else to do!

— Seven-day food and drink diary —

How to fill in your food intake diary

A column for each day of the week is provided for you to fill in. This section looks at the number of times you have foods from each of five food groups – bread and cereals; meat, fish or equivalents; dairy foods; vegetables and fruit.

Each food listed has a symbol(s) next to it to identify which food group it belongs to. It is assumed that you have had an 'average' portion of that food. All you need to do is fill in the number of servings you have at each meal.

While you could do it just for one day, the results will be much more meaningful if you do it for seven days. When you have completed your seven days, add up the number of portions for each food group and divide by seven. If you only manage to complete five days, then divide by five. You can then compare your intake with the recommended intake. Should you find you are not eating the recommended servings from a particular food group, you should make an effort to eat more foods from that group.

Each food listed belongs to a particular food group and each food group has its own symbol.

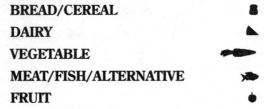

BREAD/CEREAL	
DAIRY	
VEGETABLE	
MEAT/FISH/ALTERNATIVE	
FRUIT	

The symbol alongside each food represents the amount that an 'average' portion of the food contributes to the total amount recommended for that food group. For example, 1 bowl of cereal has 1 loaf drawn next to it. This means that a bowl of cereal gives you 1 serving from the BREAD/CEREAL group.

Some foods have more than one type of symbol beside them, meaning that they are 'combination foods' and belong to more than one group. For example 1 slice of pizza has 2 loaves and 1 cheese next to it. This means that a slice of pizza gives you 2 servings from the BREAD/CEREAL group and 1 serving from the DAIRY group.

Let's go through how to fill in the diary page for one day's food and drink record:

Breakfast

2 slices toast	Enter 1 for bread in the Day 1 column. This means you get 1 loaf (1 serving) from the BREAD/CEREAL group.
1 boiled egg	Enter 1 for egg in the Day 1 column. This means you get 1 serving from the DAIRY group.

Lunch

1 ham sandwich	Enter 1 for 'filling for sandwich' and 1 for bread/cereal in the Day 1 column. This means you get 1 fish (1 MEAT serving) and 1 loaf (1 BREAD/CEREAL serving).
1 glass orange juice	Enter 1 for fruit juice. This means you get 1 apple (1 FRUIT serving).

Snack

1 pot yogurt	Enter 1 for yogurt under dairy. This means you get 1 cheese (1 DAIRY serving).

Dinner

Chicken curry	Enter 1 for meat curry. This means you get 2 fish (2 MEAT servings).
Rice	Enter 1 for rice, giving you 3 loaves (3 BREAD/CEREAL servings).
1 orange	Enter 1 for fruit. This means you get 1 apple (1 FRUIT portion).

Now, add up the symbols, calculate the totals and compare your total intake with the recommendations.

	Your total for the day	Recommended intake per day
🍞 Bread/cereal	5	5
🐟 Meat/fish/eggs	3	1–2
🧀 Dairy	2	2–3
🍅 Fruit	2	2 or more
🥕 Vegetables	0	3 or more

The seven-day diary

Bread and Breakfast Cereals	
🔲	Breakfast cereal
🔲	Bread (2 slices)/1 roll/1 chapatti
🔲	Crispbreads (2)
Dairy	
🔺	Milk (1/2 pint)/milk-shake
🔺	Milk for cereal/milk pudding
🔺	Yogurt (1 pot)
🔺	Cheese all types (1 oz)
🔲 🔲 🔺	Pizza with cheese (1 slice)
Eggs	
🔺	Egg (1)
Meat, Fish and Equivalents	
🐟 🐟	Bacon, grilled
🐟 🐟	Burger/vegetable burger
🐟 🐟	Meat/chicken, roast/grilled/fried/boiled
🐟 🐟	Meat/chicken, stew/curry
🔲 🔲 🐟 🐟	Pie/pastie
🐟	Filling for sandwich
🐟	Sauce for pasta (mince/fish)
🐟	Sausages (2 large)
🐟	Fish, grilled/boiled
🐟	Fish, stew/curry
🐟 🐟	Fish in batter/crumbs/fingers
🐟	Smoked salmon/prawns
Starchy vegetables, rice and pasta	
🔲 🐟	Beans baked/tinned/salad (1 small tin)
🔲 🐟	Peas/chickpeas/lentils
🔲 🔲 🐟	Pasta/spaghetti/noodles
🔲 🔲	Potatoes and chips/plantain/yam/cassava
🔲 🔲 🔲	Rice
Other vegetables	
🐟	Number of portions of any other veg (3–4 oz)
Fruit	
●	Number of portions of any fresh fruit/fruit juice
Total number of servings:	

Day 1	Day 2	Day 3	Day 4	Day 5	Day 6	Day 7	Total	🥛	🐟	🔺	🥖	🍎

How Ms Ideal's intake compares with the recommendations

To compare your total intake with the recommendations, fill in the table below.

	Grand total ÷ number of days recorded	Recommended intake per day
🍞 Bread/cereal		5
🐟 Meat/fish/eggs		1–2
🔺 Dairy		2–3
🍒 Fruit		2 or more
🥕 Vegetables		3 or more

Derivation of the number of servings from each group

It is only necessary to read this section if you would like more information about how the food diary works.

In our study, 'Nutrition of women in anticipation of pregnancy' (Wynn et al., 1991), the average daily intakes of 165 women who had babies in the optimum birthweight range (3.5 to 4.5 kg) were as follows:

Energy	1980 kcalories
Protein	73 g
Carbohydrate (CHO)	230 g of which 115 g was starch

For the purposes of this assessment our main concern is your intake of vitamins and minerals. We are not particularly interested in the amount of fat in the diet because foods high in fat do not generally contribute to the vitamins and minerals that we found were important when planning pregnancy.

The five food groups which would have supplied the protein and vitamins and minerals include (1) bread/cereals, (2) meat, fish or alternatives, (3) dairy foods, (4) vegetables and (5) fruit.

Using the information from the study, the number of servings from the five food groups has been worked out as follows:

Bread/cereal are good sources of starch, fibre, a variety of B vitamins and minerals.

1 bread/cereal serving (▮) = 20 g starch

The total daily amount of carbohydrate was 230 g. Of this, 115 g came from starchy foods such as bread, potatoes, rice and other cereals and the remainder came from fruit, vegetables and dairy foods.

The number of daily servings from the bread/cereal group = 115 ÷ 20 = 5–6 servings.

Meat/fish and alternatives are good sources of protein, minerals, such as iron, zinc and vitamins including B12 and B3 (niacin).

1 serving meat (3–4 oz) or equivalent (➤) = 14 g protein

The number of daily servings that came from the meat group = 1 – 2. This will provide 14–28 g of protein; the remainder will come mainly from dairy foods and cereals.

Dairy foods are a good source of protein, minerals, especially calcium, and vitamins particularly B2 (riboflavin).

1 serving of dairy foods (▲) = 14 g protein

The number of daily servings that came from dairy foods 5 2–3.

Vegetables are good sources of carbohydrate and fibre and contain a variety of vitamins and minerals, including folic acid, carotene (vitamin A) and magnesium.

1 serving of vegetables (excluding potatoes) = 5 g carbohydrate

The number of daily servings from vegetables = 3 (15 g carbohydrate).

Fruit is a good source of carbohydrate, fibre and vitamins such as vitamin C and folic acid.

1 serving of fruit = 15 g carbohydrate

The number of daily servings from fruit = 2 (30 g carbohydrate).

4

FOOD, GLORIOUS FOOD!

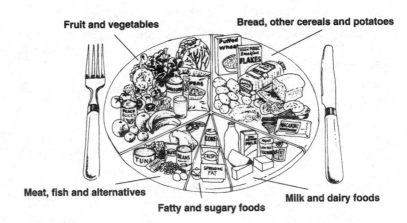

Fruit and vegetables

Bread, other cereals and potatoes

Meat, fish and alternatives

Fatty and sugary foods

Milk and dairy foods

In discussing diets and their nutritional improvement, there needs to be a balance. Food is to be enjoyed as well as to nurture our bodies. This book will have failed hopelessly if it turns the reader into a calorie-counting, vitamin-popping paranoid. Healthy eating is not incompatible with pleasurable eating, it is not a list of dos and don'ts. Choosing to eat a healthy diet is one of the most positive things you can do, not just for the baby in your future, but for your own well-being and those around you. The aim is not to leave you feeling guilty about what you eat or do not eat, but to inform and encourage you to understand the principles of healthy eating which will benefit both you and your family in the future. This book should help you feel confident in the informed choices you will make in your everyday diet.

This chapter will discuss the principles of healthy eating in terms of everyday foods, highlighting some of the issues raised in the previous chapters. Food safety will also be discussed because of the dangers of food poisoning in early pregnancy.

—— Principles of healthy eating ——

Healthy eating, it seems, is shrouded in mystique but truly, there is no magic formula and no absolute dos and don'ts.

The main concern when preparing for pregnancy, is to ensure you have an adequate supply of vitamins and minerals rather than majoring on fat or sugar. A diet which contains a lot of processed foods e.g. biscuits, cakes, confectionery, fizzy drinks, etc. will be high in fat and sugar and, as a consequence, low in vitamins and minerals.

A diet high in vitamins and minerals will contain foods from each of the five food groups mentioned in the self-assessment chapter: cereal foods, especially wholegrain varieties, lean meat or alternatives, dairy foods (remember, low-fat milk contains a much higher proportion of minerals and water-soluble vitamins per 100 kcalories than full-fat milk), vegetables and fruit.

Meal Patterns

The importance of breakfast

Whatever happened to 'three square meals a day'? It is rare for a modern family to sit down to more than one meal a day, yet breakfast is a very important meal. Not only can it be very nutritious, but it alleviates the need for biscuits, chocolate bars and other high-calorie, low-nutrient mid-morning snacks.

It has been found that school children who regularly eat breakfast cereal have significantly higher intakes of vitamins and minerals than children who do not eat cereal (Doyle et al., 1994). More importantly when planning pregnancy, it has been observed that mothers who had good-sized, healthy babies ate double the amount of breakfast cereals as mothers who had small babies (Doyle et al., 1990). There are important lessons to be learned from this:

- The mothers who ate breakfast cereals had significantly higher vitamin and mineral intakes
- The mothers who had good nutrient intakes generally had 3 meals a day
- It is difficult to meet all your nutrient requirements in anything less than three meals a day.

One of the most simple and effective ways of increasing your vitamin and mineral intakes is to have a cereal-based breakfast. If taken with milk, it will also help you to increase your calcium and protein intake; use low-fat milk if you are concerned about weight gain.

Lunch

Lunch is often a snack. Snacks can range from high-nutrient to low-nutrient content. Good, high-nutrient choices include: baked beans on granary bread, tinned salmon (or other fish)/lean meat/egg and salad sandwich made with wholemeal or granary bread, jacket potato with stir fried vegetables, homemade soup, kedgeree and salad, omelette and salad or maybe a tuna-based pasta dish with salad.

Supper

Supper is the one meal in the day when families can usually get together. It is an opportunity for a well-rounded, nutritious meal prepared from scratch. Today, with the pressure on both partners to work, we are tending towards a trend of eating out, having ready-to-eat meals or something from the local take-away. These meals are often high in calories and highly diluted in terms of nutritional content when compared to home-cooked meals using fresh ingredients.

——— Changing eating habits ———

Evolution rather than revolution!

Changing eating habits is not easy for everyone; our eating habits are often deep-rooted in our upbringing. Changing to a healthier way of eating should mean making small changes one at a time. This makes it easier to adapt and more likely to last.

Start by thinking of those five food groups – cereals/bread, meat/meat alternatives, dairy foods, vegetables and fruit. Which of these food groups are you missing out in (see Chapter 3)? How could you include more of those foods in your diet? Could you substitute some less nutritious foods for more of the foods that you wish to increase – a bowl of cereal with milk at breakfast time instead of a bar of chocolate mid-morning; a piece of fruit in place of biscuits; orange juice rather than a fizzy drink or fruit squash; a yogurt instead of a doughnut?

Variety is the spice of life

Eating a variety of foods increases the interest, enjoyment of and nutritional value of your diet. No one food contains all the nutrients needed for health, so variety in your diet is essential to create balance and obtain all the nutrients you need. Try to structure your diet thinking positively about increasing the variety of foods you eat. When did you last try a food you had not eaten before?

Despite our ready access to a variety of ethnic and interesting foods that maybe new to us, we tend to be reticent about trying new foods. Many of these are very nutritious – unusual vegetables and fruits, different pulses, unfamiliar grains; there are endless ways to combine familiar and less familiar ingredients. In recent years there have been many cookery books, magazines and TV programmes, all filled with recipes that cater for a more health-conscious audience ready to experiment.

However, whether you are an adventurous cook/eater or not, remember the five basic food groups:

Cereals and breads

Cereals are the staple diet of most cultures. Wheat provides more nourishment for the human population than any other single food. Other cereals include maize (corn), millet, oats, barley, rye and rice. Rice is considered a sign of fertility – that is why it is thrown at weddings!

Unrefined cereals are extremely nutritious; each grain is enveloped within an outer protective skin containing bran and a small area at the base of the grain: the germ. When these are processed (for instance, when making white flour) a large proportion of the bran and germ is removed. During this process most of the thiamin (B1), riboflavin (B2), niacin (B3), pyridoxine (B6), vitamin E and

Bread, other cereals and potatoes

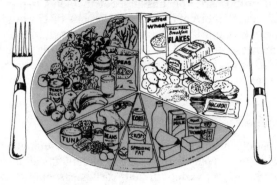

the essential fatty acids, are lost. About 20 per cent of the protein and a high proportion of the fibre is also lost during processing. Polished rice retains less than half its vitamin B6, a third of its niacin (B3), and only 20 per cent of its original thiamin (B1). The loss through processing is the reason nutritionists and dietitians constantly recommend wholemeal pasta, brown rice and wholegrain and brown breads since the whole, natural grains retain maximum nutrition.

Wholemeal bread means what it says – the whole grain. It must by law consist of 100 per cent wholemeal flour. It is nutritionally the best choice of bread.

Brown bread A wide selection of breads fall into this category, including granary and wheatgerm breads. If buying a bread that is labelled, choose the one with the highest fibre content as this will reflect the vitamin content.

White bread By law, millers have to add two B vitamins, thiamin and niacin, to the level found in brown flour (85 per cent extraction rate, i.e. 85 per cent of the grain is used and 15 per cent discarded). They also have to restore calcium and iron to the 85 per cent extraction level. White bread is lower in fibre (1.5 g per 100 g) than wholemeal (5.8 g per 100 g) or brown bread (3.5 g per 100 g), and as a nation we eat too little fibre. However, some people do prefer white bread and must not feel guilty; it is still much more nourishing than biscuits and other confectionery.

Breakfast cereals can make an important contribution, both to the fibre content of your diet and, because many cereals are fortified, to your vitamin and mineral intakes. It is a good idea to compare the nutrition labels of different cereals; for instance, a major breakfast cereal producer, Kelloggs, did some research into which of their products were most popular with women and have now fortified the three most popular cereals with extra folic acid which is so important to every woman who may become pregnant or who is already pregnant.

Meat and alternatives

Meat is a good source of animal protein as well as containing appreciable amounts of several minerals and vitamins, including iron, zinc, vitamin B12 and thiamin (B1). The nutritional content of meat is determined more by leanness because all essential nutrients will be found only in the lean part of the meat.

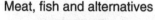

Meat, fish and alternatives

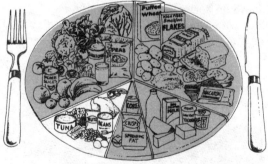

Fish is correctly perceived as a 'healthy' food. White fish such as cod is high in protein, low in fat, and a good source of B vitamins and iodine. Oily fish such as mackerel and salmon are also high in protein, B vitamins and fat-soluble vitamins A and D. In addition, oily fish are high in essential fatty acids, which are important in brain development during fetal life (Crawford et al., 1989). Studies show that women on the Faroe Islands who eat large quantities of fish have bigger babies and fewer premature babies than their Danish counterparts. This has been attributed to their intake of eicosapentanoic acid, which is an essential fatty acid found in fish. Eicosapentanoic acid inhibits the production of prostaglandins that delay the onset of labour (Olsen et al., 1986).

Eggs are rich in essential nutrients; almost all the nutrients are concentrated in the yolk for the developing chick. The yolk is also the most nourishing for us, containing protein, fat and significant amounts of vitamin A, thiamin (B1), riboflavin (B2), B12, and folic acid. An egg also contains iron, but it is poorly absorbed; the white contains protein and small amounts of vitamins and trace elements.

Eggs must be fully cooked to avoid the risk of salmonella.

Most **nuts and seeds** are high in protein and fat, the exception being chestnuts which are high in carbohydrate and low in protein and fat. Nuts and seeds are good sources of B vitamins and of iron. Because they are so high in fat, nuts are high in calories (ten large peanuts contain 100 kcalories – the equivalent of two apples or a mango). Although not regarded as an 'empty calorie snack', nuts can be a less obvious source of excess calories.

Dairy foods

Dairy foods would normally be considered under the 'Meat or alternatives' food group when considering healthy eating but, in the context of preparing for pregnancy, calcium-containing foods are very important.

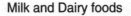

Milk and Dairy foods

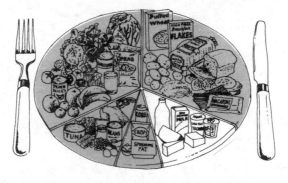

Milk is said to be the nearest thing to being a complete food. It is able to satisfy almost all our nutritional requirements except iron, vitamin D and E; but of course, full-fat milk is high in saturated fat. The saturated fat element is reduced in semi-skimmed and skimmed milk. One pint of milk (full- or low-fat) a day will provide almost all your calcium and vitamin B12, half your riboflavin (B2), 40 per cent of your protein, quarter of your zinc and 20 per cent of your magnesium and vitamin B6 requirements.

Yogurt is a fermented milk and contains all the nutrients of the milk from which it is made.

Cheese, like milk, is high in protein, calcium and vitamin B2. Some soft ripened cheeses such as Brie or Camembert may contain listeria, and for this reason the government has recommended that pregnant women should avoid them (DoH/MAFF, 1992).

Fruit and vegetables

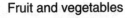
Fruit and vegetables

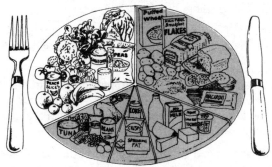

Vegetables are a very important source of vitamins, minerals and fibre and an essential part of a healthy diet.

Dried beans and peas Vegetables such as red kidney beans, black-eyed beans, chickpeas and lentils are edible seeds. They are nourishing, inexpensive and versatile. These vegetables complement stews very well and can be used to replace some of the more expensive meat component. While they are rich sources of protein as well as starch, they also contain fibre, B vitamins and essential minerals. With their content and versatility they are an excellent food for vegetarians.

Green leafy vegetables, especially the darker green varieties such as spinach, spring greens and purple sprouting broccoli, contain significant amounts of folic acid, vitamin C and carotene (vitamin A) as well as iron and other trace elements. All green vegetables should be lightly cooked in order to preserve the nutrients and retain their taste and texture.

Root vegetables, especially the yellow varieties like carrots, are rich in carotene and are often good sources of thiamin (Vitamin B1).

Potatoes are often falsely thought of as fattening. Four-fifths of the weight of a potato is water and if eaten without fat, the energy density is relatively low. Potatoes provide us with significant amounts of protein, fibre, vitamin C and vitamin B6; they are not a concentrated source of these nutrients, but because we eat them regularly and in reasonable amounts they are a significant provider. A high proportion of the nutrients are just under the skin and therefore more nutritious when eaten with the skin, or at least cooked with their skin before peeling.

Fruit, with all its shapes, colours, flavours and smells, appeals to all our senses, yet in Britain we eat less than most other European countries.

Citrus fruits such as oranges and grapefruit are particularly high in vitamin C, as are strawberries, blackcurrants, kiwi fruit and guavas. Yellow fruits like apricots, peaches and mangoes are good sources of carotene; the precursor of vitamin A.

Dried fruits are a good source of iron and other trace elements but because we do not eat these in appreciable amounts they cannot be considered an important source in most people's diet.

Folic acid is found in moderate amounts in clementines, satsumas, oranges, blackberries and raspberries.

High-energy, low-nutrient foods

What do biscuits, cakes, sweets, chocolate, sugar, jam, pastry, fizzy drinks and crisps have in common? They all contain lots of sugar and/or fat and very few vitamins and minerals. Eating too much of these foods will take the place of other good, nutrient-rich foods. This satisfaction of your appetite is at the cost of your vitamin and mineral requirements.

These high-energy, low-nutrient foods must be regarded as 'occasional' foods – not as a regular feature in your diet – and should not

Fatty and sugary foods

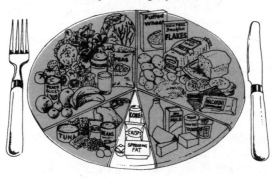

take the place of the foods from the five food groups mentioned above.

Butter, margarines, low-fat spreads, cooking fats and oils are also high in calories and low in nutrients, so should be used moderately. If you use margarine or oil, choose one that is high in 'polyunsaturates' such as sunflower, corn or soya.

--- **Food safety** ---

Pregnancy will alter your immune response making you more vulnerable to infections which can be transmitted to your unborn baby. This is particularly important in the early stages of your pregnancy because the immune system of the fetus is not sufficiently well developed to fight infection. Care in preparing food is therefore very important if you are to avoid the unpleasant consequences of food poisoning.

The most common form of food poisoning in the home is caused by contamination with the bacteria, salmonella. Foods most commonly associated with food poisoning include undercooked poultry and eggs, meat products, shellfish and soft-rinded cheeses. Food poisoning is more common in warm weather when the bacteria can multiply very quickly; keeping foods properly refrigerated reduces bacterial activity.

It is sensible to take simple precautions to reduce the risk to you and your baby. Here is a list of tips on general food safety:

Hygiene

- Wash your hands before and after handling food, especially after touching raw poultry and meat
- Keep food surfaces in the kitchen clean and discourage cats from walking over them
- Use one board and knife for preparing raw poultry and meat and another for other foods. Wash them thoroughly after use.

Food safety

- After a shopping trip, don't leave food in your car for any longer than is essential, especially in warm weather
- Don't eat food which has passed its 'use by' date
- Cook eggs, poultry and meat thoroughly
- When reheating food, make sure it is piping hot all the way through.

In the fridge

- Keep your fridge between 0–5°C
- Keep raw food away from cooked food
- Store raw poultry and meat on the lowest shelf in the fridge to avoid them dripping onto other foods
- Defrost food fully before cooking, especially poultry.

Foods to avoid when planning pregnancy

- Soft, ripe cheeses such as Camembert and Brie
- Raw or undercooked meats
- Liver
- Raw eggs.

Safety with pets

- Wash your hands after handling pets
- Keep pets off surfaces where you prepare food
- Wear rubber gloves when cleaning cat-litter trays
- Wear rubber gloves when gardening.

5

IMPROVING YOUR LIFESTYLE

The use of tobacco, alcohol, illicit drugs and, possibly, high intakes of caffeine, have important health implications, not just for you but also for your unborn child.

Smoking

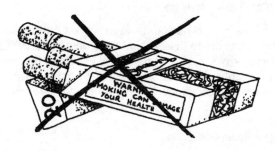

The harmful effects of tobacco on pregnancy outcome were first suggested in the mid-nineteenth century, when doctors observed that women who worked in tobacco factories were more prone to miscarriage.

The harmful effects of smoking to the unborn child are impossible to dispute in spite of the echoes 'My friend smoked 20 a day during her pregnancy and her baby was OK.' The fact is the friend was taking a risk with her unborn baby's health, and no one is in a position to predict the outcome while exposing their baby to risk of damage.

We know that smoking makes it more difficult to conceive, with both partners compromising the chances of achieving pregnancy. There is a higher percentage of infertility among couples who smoke (Chamberlain, 1990). Smoking impairs a woman's capacity to produce a fertilisable egg; advice following a study on smoking and reduced fertility was that 'women who were unable to conceive should stop smoking, especially before treatment with in-vitro fertilisation' (Rosevear et al., 1992). Smoking will also reduce her partner's ability to produce healthy sperm.

In the United States, smoking during pregnancy has been identified as being the single most important preventable determinant of low birthweight and perinatal death. As well as infertility, other associations that have been found between smoking and pregnancy outcome are: (a) miscarriage, (b) premature delivery, (c) low birthweight, (d) physical abnormalities at birth, (e) stillbirth and death within the first month of life. There can be no doubt that the baby of smoking parents is disadvantaged even before it is conceived, and parents-to-be should be aware of these dangers (Mosher and Pratt, 1987).

Smoking and miscarriage

Lower levels of certain hormones in expectant mothers who smoke have led researchers to believe that these lower levels of hormones is one reason why smoking results in ill effects to the unborn baby. This is especially the case in relation to miscarriage, which is known to be influenced by hormonal changes (Bernstein et al., 1989).

Smoking and birthweight

One of the most important consequences of women smoking during pregnancy is that their unborn babies do not grow as big as babies of non-smoking mothers. There is a direct relationship between maternal smoking and birthweight – the higher the number of cigarettes smoked, the lower the birthweight is likely to be. It is therefore still beneficial to cut down if you are unable to stop altogether. Babies born to mothers who smoke are between 150 and 250 g (5–9 oz) lighter, or 8 to 9 g for each cigarette smoked on a daily basis, than babies of mothers who do not smoke (Lincoln, 1986) and they double their risk of having a low-birthweight baby.

Smoking and birth abnormalities

Mothers who smoke during pregnancy are 60 per cent more likely to give birth to babies with a cleft palate or hair lip than women who do not smoke during their pregnancy (Khoury et al., 1989).

Smoking and intellectual attainment

Mothers who smoke during and after pregnancy have babies with slightly smaller heads on average than the babies of non-smokers. Although the heads are only slightly smaller, head size at birth has been closely linked with brain development. So maternal smoking could influence the mental abilities of their children (Elwood et al., 1987). These findings are supported by a number of studies which have reported a slower intellectual maturity in children whose mothers smoked during pregnancy. One study showed that on average, children of women who did not smoke during pregnancy attained higher educational qualifications by the age of 23 than those whose mothers did smoke (Fogelman et al., 1988).

Influence of father's smoking

Stopping or reducing the number of cigarettes smoked should not just apply to the mother. There is evidence from a large study in Germany which found that smoking by the father, when the mother did not smoke, was associated with an increased incidence of miscarriage, premature births and low birthweight (Koller, 1983).

Following birth, children of smoking parents are more likely to suffer with ill health, having higher rates of respiratory problems and a greater risk of cot death in the first year of life. A major cause of wheezy bronchitis in infants is passive smoking (Newspeil et al., 1989).

Giving up

Giving up smoking is very difficult, but more people succeed when planning or during pregnancy than at other times. Most women are motivated by the fact that they wish to have a healthy baby and stopping smoking is a very positive step they can take to look after their baby while still in the womb. However, the support of each partner to the other is crucial when trying to give up.

The technique used to stop smoking will differ from person to person and for those who feel they would benefit from outside support, there are a number of organisations who can help. Your local Citizens' Advice Bureau should be able to provide the names and addresses of these groups. Two such groups include:

For written advice   Action on Smoking and Health (ASH)
109 Gloucester Place
London W1H 3PH
Telephone 0171 935 3519

For counselling   Telephone **Quitline** on 0171 487 3000

Alcohol

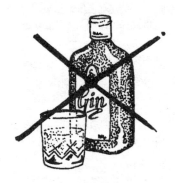

From ancient times there have been warnings about drinking alcohol during pregnancy. Heavy drinking is recognised as potentially damaging to the unborn baby, especially early in pregnancy. In 1759, the London College of Surgeons attempted to persuade the government to raise taxes on gin in order to make it less available to expectant mothers. Today the United States Surgeon General recommends that women who are pregnant, or who are considering pregnancy, abstain from alcoholic drinks. The British Royal College of Obstetricians and Gynaecologists also recommends that women avoid alcohol during pregnancy.

Children suffering from mental defects, unusual facial characteristics and growth retardation have frequently been observed in alcoholic families. Children born to heavy-drinking mothers are now recognised as suffering from Fetal Alcohol Syndrome.

Alcohol crosses the placenta and can build up to toxic levels, the effects of which are most severe in early pregnancy during rapid cell division. Alcohol abuse will also affect the fetus indirectly through its effect on maternal nutrition. It is sometimes described as an anti-nutrient because its consumption can lead to malabsorption, poor utilisation or increased urinary excretion of essential nutrients, in particular zinc, thiamin, vitamin A and folic acid, all of which are important in pregnancy.

A safe level of alcohol has not yet been defined in relation to pregnancy and the available evidence is inconsistent. A study of 952 pregnancies in Dundee found that alcohol consumption of less than 100 g (ten standard drinks) per week produced no measurable adverse effects (Sulaiman et al., 1988). Another study on more than 30,000 pregnancies found that there was an increased risk of growth retardation associated with one or two drinks a day, even after adjusting for other important risk factors such as smoking (Mills et al., 1984).

This does not mean the expectant mother should spend her pregnancy racked with worry about the drinks she had before she found she was pregnant. Many women have unwittingly indulged in an episode or two of heavy drinking before they discovered they were pregnant, without there being any ill effects.

Both partners should be aware that alcohol is potentially damaging to their unborn baby, the consequences of which may be more subtle than would be detected at birth. The best advice is probably to err on the side of caution – if you are trying to conceive, stop drinking alcohol or at least avoid excessive amounts, as adverse effects to the embryo could occur before pregnancy is confirmed. It is wise to keep consumption prior to conception to no more than one unit of alcohol per day. A unit is equivalent to one glass of wine, $\frac{1}{2}$ pint beer or one pub measure of spirits.

Cutting down

For some people, alcohol is just an occasional social habit; for others, it may be an addiction, and cutting down to no more than one unit a day can be difficult, especially if their partner is a regular drinker. It is not necessary to stop the habit of 'drinking', just to having alcohol in your drink. Have your drink at your normal 'cocktail hour' or with your meal, but have a juice spritzer (half fruit juice, half sparkling water), grape juice or a low- or non-alcoholic wine or beer.

Caffeine

People have enjoyed caffeine-containing beverages from ancient times, but concerns have been voiced about the health effects of caffeine, found mainly in coffee, tea and cola drinks. Information about the influence of caffeine on birth outcome is very limited and there is no evidence that caffeine causes birth defects in humans.

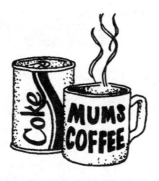

There may, however, be a link between caffeine consumption and miscarriage. The Journal of the American Medical Association reported a study (Infante-Rivard et al., 1993) which found the risk of miscarriage doubled in women who drank two or three cups of ground coffee or its equivalent in other caffeine containing drinks:

AVERAGE CAFFEINE CONTENT OF DRINKS

1 cup of ground coffee	115 mg
1 cup of instant coffee	65 mg
1 cup of tea	40 mg
1 can of cola	33 mg

Of course, as with all situations in life, one woman's tolerance level to caffeine will be much higher than another's. The best advice is to limit coffee and caffeine-containing products, possibly to four cups/drinks a day.

--------------------- # Drugs ---------------------

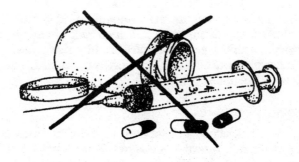

Many drugs are potentially harmful, whether they are socially acceptable or otherwise. Certain generalisations can be made about all drugs before and during pregnancy:

- all drugs should be avoided unless clearly needed
- when using drugs, whether prescribed or self-administered, always ask the doctor or pharmacist about the possible harm to the embryo or fetus
- if you use drugs for a medical condition, do not discontinue without discussing with your doctor – remember, your baby's health depends on your health.

Self-administered drugs/pills

Of the many drugs available over the counter, few will be harmful to the unborn child but it is wise to consult your pharmacist before buying any drugs.

Prescribed drugs

Not all prescribed drugs are potentially harmful to the unborn baby, and as long as your doctor is aware that you are attempting to become pregnant he or she will weigh up whether the benefit derived from a drug outweighs any potential risk. Remember, however, that in the early stages you may not be aware of your pregnancy so you should inform your doctor if there is a possibility that you could be pregnant.

Street Drugs

Heroin

Heroin and other opiates are less commonly used in the UK; but for those who do use them, there is a high risk of poor outcome of pregnancy, including perinatal mortality (the risk is two-and-a-half times higher), premature delivery (risk twice as high) and growth retardation (five times greater risk).

Cocaine

Cocaine or crack abuse is associated with a higher risk of miscarriage, prematurity, growth retardation, brain lesions and physical malformation. Cocaine-exposed babies are eight times more likely to be of low birthweight (Chamberlain, 1990). Babies born to cocaine-addicted mothers usually suffer withdrawal symptoms when born.

Marijuana

The use of marijuana, or pot, is more common. Regular use may increase the risk of premature labour and maternal weight gain can be lower. As with other drugs, it is difficult to separate the effects of the drug from other inter-related social factors such as smoking, alcohol and poor nutrition. Its effects on the unborn baby are equivocal but the baby may suffer withdrawal symptoms causing increased irritability and agitation in the first few days after birth.

– Environmental and work hazards –

While most jobs present little threat to pregnancy, working conditions in some industries can expose employees to hazardous

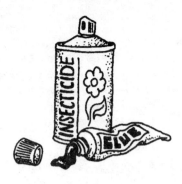

substances. In general, however, there is great concern in business, agriculture, waste disposal sites and other places of work, not to expose employees to toxic substances, especially before and during pregnancy.

Nevertheless, environmental pollutants are real, and they do occur both in the work place and in the home. Fumes, solvents, some metals such as mercury, and chemicals such as those used in the manufacture of plastics and agricultural chemicals, are all possible causes of infertility, miscarriage and poor outcome of pregnancy. It should be remembered that habits such as maternal smoking and alcohol consumption are generally thought to be more harmful for the unborn child than exposure to occupational hazards. However, it is wise to avoid any unnecessary exposure to potentially toxic substances, whether work-related or not.

In men, toxic agents can cause decreased libido and impotence and in women, menstrual disorders, infertility, miscarriage, growth retardation and fetal abnormalities. Toxic agents may be physical, biological or chemical:

Physical

Radiation, most commonly experienced through X-rays, is known to be harmful to reproduction and anyone who may be pregnant or who is pregnant should avoid exposure to it. Attention is usually drawn to avoiding radiation exposure to anyone known to be pregnant, but the fetus is most vulnerable during the early stages, before pregnancy may have been discovered.

Biological

These can be an occupational hazard, as in the case of hospital workers in contact with infectious patients, those working with children, farmers and butchers. Bacterial infections include listeria and salmonella. Viruses include rubella, measles, mumps, herpes and cytomegalovirus.

Chemical

Exposure to chemicals known to be reproductive toxins include:

- metals, such as lead, cadmium and mercury
- solvents (dry-cleaning fluids and paint strippers)
- pesticides, including organophosphates
- insecticides, such as dieldran
- pollutants, such as PCB (polychlorinated biphenyls) used in the manufacture of plastics.

The Health and Safety Commission has set out proposals to implement the health and safety provisions of the EC Directive on pregnant workers (1994). These guidelines include assessment of chemical, physical and biological agents and industrial processes considered hazardous to pregnant women, women who have recently given birth and women who are breast-feeding.

If you are worried about toxic substances at work, consult your company's health and safety officer; if no one is available for such consultation, contact the Health and Safety Executive in London, telephone number 0171 229 3456.

Exercise

The specific effects of strenuous exercise around the time of conception have not been fully determined. Women who take part in competitive endurance sports can experience menstrual irregularity, which may cause difficulties in conceiving. There is no evidence, however, that menstrual disorders caused by physical activity are permanently harmful for the woman athlete. Women who are very lean will usually regain regular periods by increasing their body weight.

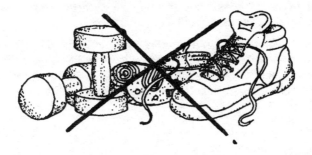

High body temperatures (hyperthermia) through vigorous exercising may have harmful effects on the unborn baby, especially in the early weeks of pregnancy (Bullard, 1981). It is therefore advisable to reduce the level of strenuous exercise from the time you are likely to have conceived.

For those who have established exercise routines, as long as there is no risk of hyperthermia, they should continue to enjoy their exercise.

The American College of Obstetrics and Gynecologists have suggested that vigorous exercise should not be undertaken in certain circumstances. These include having had three or more miscarriages or having experienced in a previous pregnancy: cervical incompetence; premature labour; intrauterine growth retardation or placenta previal (may have caused bleeding in previous pregnancy).

If you want to continue any form of strenuous exercise, it would be wise to discuss this with your doctor, before you conceive.

Stress

Stress is often thought to be responsible for problems that occur in pregnancy, including infertility, miscarriage and congenital abnormalities. However, researchers who have attempted to assess the effects of stress in pregnancy admit that there is little firm evidence to support any of these claims. It is very difficult to isolate stress *per se* from associated factors. It may, for example, be that poverty is a risk factor for poor outcome of pregnancy, partly because of the high levels of stress associated with being poor.

The conclusion of one large study carried out in the mid 1980s was that psycho-social stress, measured by adverse life events, anxiety, depression, poor social support and perceived income difficulties, had little relation to birth outcome (Brooke et al., 1989).

6

A GENERAL HEALTH CHECK

It is often easier to resolve health problems during the planning stages of pregnancy, so if you are worried about any aspect of your general health, seek advice from your doctor or the practice nurse at your doctor's surgery. A short checklist of common problems that should be attended to includes:

- Rubella, check you are immune to rubella (German measles) – see below for more information
- Varicose veins and foot problems, such as corns or verrucae – the extra weightload of pregnancy could cause you additional discomfort
- Haemorrhoids
- Inverted nipples
- Bladder problems, such as a recurrent discharge or infection
- Bowel problems, such as constipation
- Dental and gum problems.

Chronic illness

The majority of women who are pregnant or hoping to become pregnant are in the 16–34 age range, a time when most people are fit and healthy. However, even in this age group, a few women are unfortunate enough to suffer from chronic health problems and may be concerned how their medical condition may affect their unborn child, particularly if the mother is taking medication. Pregnancy and the possibility of causing a deterioration in her own health is likely to be a further concern.

In order to understand what to expect from the interaction of pregnancy and a pre-existing disorder, it is important to consult your doctor in the planning stages of pregnancy, particularly if you are suffering from any of the following:

- Hormonal disorders such as diabetes or an overactive thyroid
- Respiratory disorders including asthma, tuberculosis or cystic fibrosis
- Neurological disorders such as multiple sclerosis or epilepsy
- Heart and circulatory problems such as raised blood pressure
- Kidney disease
- AIDS (Acquired Immune Deficiency Syndrome).

Knowledge in all of these areas of medicine are advancing rapidly and you should not rely on the information of library books written five years ago, or advice from well-meaning but poorly informed friends or relatives. Do see your doctor who may refer you to a specialist for assessment. The specialist will be able to inform you of any risks to your own health and that of your planned baby. You will then be able to make an informed choice and act accordingly.

Pre-pregnancy weight

Your pre-pregnancy weight has a direct impact on the birthweight of your baby. A useful method of estimating the risk to health and reproductive success is the Body Mass Index (BMI). This is an index of a person's weight in relation to their height. It is calculated by dividing your weight (in kilograms) by the square of your height (in metres):

$$\text{Body Mass Index} = \text{weight (kg)} \div \text{height}^2 \text{ (metres)}$$

Weight in pounds (1 stone = 14 lb) can be converted to kilograms by multiplying pounds by 0.4536. Height in inches can be converted to metres by multiplying inches by 0.0254.

For example, if you are 10 stone (10×14 lb = 140 lb $\times$ 0.4536 = 63.5 kg) and 5 ft 5 in (65 in $\times$ 0.0254 = 1.65 metres), your BMI would be $63.5 \div 1.65^2 = 23.3$.

The normal BMI gradations are:

BMI

Underweight	=	less than 20
Acceptable weight	=	20–24.9
Overweight	=	25–29.9
Fat	=	30–39.9
Very fat	=	greater than 40

A BMI of 23 to 24 is considered good for general health, fertility and for birthweight (Wynn and Wynn, 1990).

Underweight

Low BMI, which in many cases may reflect nutritional status, is known to increase the risk of low birthweight. It is also an important cause of amenorrhoea (absence of menstruation).

A study of women who failed to conceive while constantly practising weight control showed that when they returned to a normal eating pattern, fertility was restored in 19 out of 26 women (Bates et al., 1982).

Another study of underweight women and pregnancy outcome showed that underweight women (BMI below 19.1 kg/m^2) had a threefold increased risk of having a low-birthweight baby (Van der Spuy et al., 1988). Underweight women in whom ovulation had to be induced, had an even higher risk of having a low-birthweight baby.

If you are planning pregnancy and are underweight, it is best to postpone conception until you achieve normal body weight or until you have made a concentrated effort to eat very well i.e. a high-calorie, high-vitamin and high-mineral intake for at least three to six months.

Overweight

Women who are overweight (BMIs above 30 kg/m^2) when they conceive are more likely to face pregnancy problems such as hypertension, pre-eclampsia and gestational diabetes.

It is best therefore to try to lose excess weight well in advance of your planned pregnancy, allowing two or three months of less rigorous and well-planned eating before conception, that will restrict only the high calorie, low nutrient foods (as in 'occasional foods' mentioned in Chapter 4). In that way you are unlikely to compromise your vitamin and mineral status at the time you conceive.

The older mother

The percentage of births to women aged 35 or over is increasing for a number of reasons, such as career priorities, financial concerns, or late or second marriages.

It is generally agreed that the ability to conceive diminishes with advancing age and that women who give birth in their mid-thirties, or above, have an increased risk of problems such as miscarriage, high blood pressure, pre-eclampsia and low birthweight. The incidence of chromosomal abnormalities such as Down's syndrome also increases with age. However, statistics comparing the outcome of pregnancy of older with younger mothers may be unduly alarming and although there are increased risks, the vast majority of older mothers will have normal, healthy babies. Most hospitals routinely offer older mothers amniocentesis or a triple blood test early in pregnancy so that abnormalities can be detected, and parents can then decide what action to take.

If you wish to postpone pregnancy, it is probably best to postpone it until your late twenties rather than your thirties. In doing so, you are unlikely to compromise your chances of conceiving and help to avoid pregnancy problems that occur with advancing years.

Infections

Pregnancy alters a woman's immune response and this may lead to infection which can be transmitted to the unborn child. In the early part of pregnancy (before 16 weeks) the fetus is most susceptible to infection, which can have serious effects.

It is much better to prevent an infection rather than to have to treat one, and attempts to conceive should be delayed if a course of treatment has been prescribed by your doctor. It is advisable for both partners not to use drugs (both prescribed and non-prescribed) during the vulnerable time around conception. For instance, antibiotics can interfere with sperm production. Human sperm take a period of 12 to 13 weeks to develop and it may take three months to eliminate damaged sperm and recover normal fertility following a course of antibiotics.

Rubella

German measles (rubella) is a relatively inconsequential illness to have as a child or even as an adult but is a potentially serious threat to the unborn child. Rubella can also be the cause of miscarriage and stillbirth. German measles caught by a mother during her pregnancy, particularly during the first three months of pregnancy, can have devastating consequences to her unborn child, causing abnormalities of the heart, brain and intestinal tract. Rubella is still thought to be responsible for two to three per cent of mental retardation at birth in the UK (Ho-Yen and Joss, 1988).

As part of pre-pregnancy planning, it is very important to check if you are immune to rubella **before** you become pregnant. This is easily done by a blood test to check rubella antibody levels; if the level of immunity is low, your doctor may give you a vaccination to stimulate resistance. This should be done at least three months prior to anticipated pregnancy.

Girls are now routinely vaccinated against rubella at school, so you may have been already vaccinated. If so, or if you have had German measles, you are probably immune to it. However, no one can be absolutely sure of immunity and it is safer to be checked by your doctor.

Teachers of small children, and childminders, are particularly vulnerable to rubella as childhood is the most common time for this infection. It is therefore especially important for this group of women to check their immune status.

– Food- and animal-borne infections –

Toxoplasmosis, listeriosis and salmonella infections are all caused by contact with infected food or animals. While they are relatively rare, it is sensible to take simple precautions to avoid them and so reduce any risk to you and your baby. You will find more detailed advice about safe food preparation in Chapter 4.

Toxoplasmosis

Toxoplasmosis is an infection caused by a parasite. Like German measles, it is not usually dangerous and may even go unnoticed in the healthy adult or child, or it can sometimes cause flu-like symptoms. However, in rare incidences, infection early in pregnancy can cause miscarriage or brain damage to the baby.

According to the Toxoplasmosis Trust, three out of ten people will have been infected by the age of 30 and if you have had toxoplasmosis you will be immune for life. Testing for immunity is not carried out routinely in this country but a blood test can identify whether or not you are immune. You can approach your GP for such a test before you become pregnant. If the tests suggest you are not immune, you will need to take a more cautious approach to the avoidance of infection.

Toxoplasmosis is caught from eating raw or undercooked meats, unpasteurised goat's milk and milk products, and unwashed fruit and vegetables. Animals such as cats, which hunt their prey or scavenge for food, are likely to be a source of infection and can pass it on in faeces.

Avoiding toxoplasmosis

Meat

Wash your hands thoroughly after handling raw meat. Do not eat raw or undercooked meat.

Vegetables and fruit

Remove any soil, which can carry the infection if fouled by cats, and wash carefully.

Gardening

Wear rubber gloves when gardening to avoid soil-borne contamination.

Goat's milk

If you drink goat's milk, it should be pasteurised or ultra-heat treated (UHT).

Cats

Avoid, or wear rubber gloves when handling litter trays. Always wash your hands after handling cats or kittens.

Sheep

Sheep can also be infected with toxoplasmosis. If you live or work on a farm and are pregnant, or likely to become so (remember you may not know you are pregnant in the early stages), you should avoid helping with lambing or milking ewes.

If you would like more information about toxoplasmosis, contact the Toxoplasmosis Trust, 61–71 Collier Street, London N1 9BE.

Listeriosis

Food poisoning from listeria infection can also result in miscarriage, stillbirth or severe illness in the newborn child. Although a rare disease, it is sensible to avoid foods that are major sources of the listeria bacteria during the planning stages and early pregnancy:

Soft, ripe cheeses

Cheeses such as Brie, Camembert and soft blue-veined varieties have been found to contain high levels of listeria and should be avoided throughout pregnancy, especially the early stages. Cheeses that are safe to eat and enjoy are hard cheeses, processed cheese, cheese spreads and cottage cheese.

Sheep

As with toxoplasmosis, sheep can be infected with listeria. If you are pregnant or planning to become pregnant and live in an agricultural environment, it is best to avoid helping with lambing or milking ewes.

Pâté

High levels of listeria have been found in some pâtés so they are best avoided. You are also advised to avoid liver pâté because of its high levels of vitamin A.

Cook-chilled and ready-to-eat meals

These can contain the listeria bacteria, particularly ready-to-eat poultry. These meals should be thoroughly reheated before eating. Inadequate refrigeration can seriously increase the risk of listeriosis.

Salmonella

Salmonella is one of the commonest causes of food poisoning. Although it may not have any direct effect on your unborn child, it is sensible to avoid the distress caused by severe vomiting and diarrhoea.

Eggs

Because of the risk of acquiring salmonella from raw eggs, the Department of Health advises everyone to avoid eating raw eggs and dishes which contain uncooked eggs such as mousse. If you are pregnant or likely to become pregnant, the advice is to eat only eggs which have been thoroughly cooked, i.e. where both yolk and white are solid.

Poultry

Raw poultry and meat may contain the salmonella bacteria. The bacteria are destroyed when exposed to high temperatures so meat, especially poultry, should be thoroughly cooked.

When storing before cooking, care should be taken not to allow these items to touch other foods or to drip onto food stored below them in the fridge.

Chopping boards should be washed thoroughly after contact with raw chicken or other raw meats. It is best to have a separate chopping board for preparing raw meat and poultry in order to avoid cross-infection.

Wash your hands after handling raw meat and poultry.

—— Sexually transmitted diseases ——

The following sexually transmitted diseases in either partner can affect the unborn child: herpes, cytomegalovirus, chlamydia, human papilloma virus, gonorrhoea, syphilis, hepatitis B, and human immunodeficiency virus (HIV).

In recent years there has been a switch in the prevalence of syphilis and gonorrhoea, which are relatively easy to diagnose, to much smaller organisms such as chlamydia and the mycoplasmas, papilloma and herpes viruses, viral hepatitis and HIV.

Herpes

There are two types of herpes, Type I and Type II. Type I is associated with cold sores or blisters around the mouth. Type II is associated with a genital infection which is of concern during pregnancy.

Primary infection with genital herpes early in pregnancy is associated with an increased risk of miscarriage, low birthweight and congenital malformations.

If either you or your partner has a history of recurrent herpes it is advisable to discuss it with your doctor. It is recommended that your partner use a latex condom during intercourse thoughout pregnancy. This may help to reduce recurrent episodes of herpes.

It will be advisable to have a cervical smear test in the last four weeks of pregnancy. If the virus is active near the time of the expected date of delivery, cesarean delivery may be recommended to prevent infecting the baby by delivery through the birth canal.

If you have had genital herpes you should have regular cervical smears, as the infection may encourage the development of cervical cancer.

Chlamydia

Chlamydia trachomatis infection is reported to be the most common sexually transmitted disease in developed countries today (Reid, 1990). This infection is important because of the potentially damaging effects on the newborn. Babies can acquire chlamydial infection through contact with maternal genital secretions during delivery. Chlamydial infection is the commonest cause of conjunctivitis in the newborn. It has also been associated with an increased risk of prematurity and low birthweight.

Screening for chlamydial infection should be considered in the planning stages of pregnancy for women who have a history of pelvic inflammatory disease, multiple partners or a sexually transmitted disease.

The use of latex condoms is recommended if infected until the course of treatment has been completed.

Pregnancy should be delayed for about three to four months after prescribed treatment.

Human Papilloma Virus (HPV)

Prevalence of HPV has been increasing in Europe, with a reported higher incidence than for herpes virus in England and Wales. HPV proliferates during pregnancy and the genital lesions can be so extensive that cesarean delivery is necessary to prevent maternal trauma during delivery. These lesions may result in viral transmission to the fetus, causing recurrent childhood respiratory infections.

In the pre-pregnancy period, lesions can be treated by a variety of techniques and medications, but treatment with vaginal antiseptic creams may be necessary during pregnancy since the chances of recurrence or continued growth are high.

Cytomegalovirus (CMV)

CMV is a member of the herpes group of infections and is thought to be the cause of ten per cent of congenital mental retardation in the UK (Hurley, 1983). Most newborns are infected at the time of birth through exposure to contaminated maternal blood, urine, or cervical or breast secretions.

Occupations where risk of exposure to the virus is greatest include childminders, nursery teachers and paediatric nurses, who should be scrupulous about washing hands after each contact with body secretions or the handling and disposal of used nappies.

Viral Hepatitis

Only Hepatitis B virus (HBV) has been documented as transmissible to the fetus. HBV infection is a blood-borne and sexually transmitted disease. This disease occurs predominantly in homosexual men, intravenous drug users, and those who have acquired the disease through heterosexual contacts.

Pregnant women who have the active disease and those who are chronic carriers can transmit the infection to their fetus. Most infants who are infected become permanent carriers and have a 25 per cent risk of dying from a liver-related disease (Beasley, 1983).

HIV/AIDS

AIDS is a major public health problem. HIV (Human Immunodeficiency Virus) is usually transmitted sexually: it is also transmitted through infected blood and blood products, and the sharing of needles among infected drug users. Transmission to the infant can occur *in utero* or during delivery. Studies indicate transmission rates from mother to baby being 30–65 per cent (Wang and Smaill, 1989). The infected newborn may be born with recurrent bacterial infections, persistent or recurrent thrush, and a failure to thrive.

Pregnancy may exacerbate HIV associated diseases, so it is best to seek medical advice prior to conceiving.

Gonorrhoea

Gonorrhoea is a bacterial infection that may go undetected in as many as half of all infected women. Screening for gonorrhoea before pregnancy is therefore recommended for anyone who has had multiple sexual partners, or those who have a history of sexually transmitted disease, because of the severe effects it can have on both the mother and her baby. The most common infection in newborns is conjunctivitis.

Chlamydia infection is common in those who have or have had gonorrhoea; if there is a history of gonorrhoea it is safer to be checked for chlamydia too.

Gonorrhoea is treated with antibiotics and it is important not to have any sexual contact until the infection has been successfully treated.

Syphilis

Syphilis is another bacterial infection and is a potentially serious but rare disease. Mothers with untreated syphilis can pass the infection to their baby at any stage and infected mothers have an increased risk of miscarriage and pre-term delivery.

Syphilis can be treated with antibiotics. Sexual relations must be avoided until treatment has been completed and clearance confirmed.

7

OBSTETRIC HISTORY

——— Oral contraception ———

Oral contraception can be either a combination of oestrogen and progesterone, which is called the pill, or it may be progesterone only, called the mini-pill. The latter contraceptive is often prescribed if a woman is breast-feeding or if she is a heavy smoker. It may also be prescribed if she is very overweight.

Hormones levels return to normal very quickly (within three or four days) after stopping oral contraceptives but the biological effects on ovulation can remain for as long as six weeks.

The customary advice for women seeking to become pregnant used to be to stop taking the pill two or three months prior to the time they wanted to conceive, and use some other form of contraception in the meantime. The Family Planning Association now advises those planning pregnancy to wait until they have had one normal period after stopping the pill. This is usually within four to six weeks but for some may take longer. Meanwhile, you should use an alternative method of contraception. For further advice you may contact the helpline for The Family Planning Association, telephone 0171 636 7866.

There have been reports that prolonged use of the contraceptive pill may reduce blood levels of zinc and water soluble vitamins including thiamin, riboflavin, B6, B12, folic acid and vitamin C. This is unlikely to be the case for women who have a good diet but such drug/nutrient interactions may be of relevance to those whose diets are poor, with borderline nutrient intakes. In such cases it may be advisable to use alternative methods of contraception for three or four months before trying to conceive in order to build up nutrient reserves.

Birth spacing

Close birth spacing increases the risk of miscarriage, lower birth-weights and birth abnormalities and, in particular, damage to the nervous system. These adverse effects are linked to what is called the *puerperium*, a period of time which lasts from birth to six to eight weeks after delivery when the reproductive organs are returning to normal, hormones levels are readjusting and your nutritional status is recovering from depletion caused by the first pregnancy.

During the latter part of pregnancy the placenta acts as a scavenging pump, extracting many nutrients from your blood and pumping them at higher concentrations into the fetus. Numerous studies have shown that many mothers suffer from vitamin deficiencies at the end of pregnancy and may take as long as two years to recover (Wynn, 1987). It has also been shown that it can take up to two years after pregnancy before pre-pregnancy iron levels (serum ferritin) are regained (Worthington-Roberts et al., 1989). A British study found 25 per cent of women suffered from quite severe folic acid deficiency at the end of pregnancy (Chanarin, 1979). These low levels of nutrients found in the mother following pregnancy are why close birth spacing should be avoided.

Australian studies have shown that 36 per cent of all cases of neural tube defects were born within one year of a previous birth; neural tube defects are known to be associated with poor maternal nutrition and with folic acid deficiency.

A study of nearly 1700 nine-year-old Chinese children showed that less serious, but none the less important, consequences of close birth spacing can be detrimental to school performance (Martin, 1978).

Although it is unwise to extrapolate findings from animal experiments to what may happen in humans, it may be useful to make general observations which are consistent through species similar in origin. In farm animals, close birth spacing has great economic importance and there are obvious commercial incentives for over-coming any undesirable consequences. This has led farmers, who recognise the association between close birth spacing and nutrition-al depletion, to provide excellent nutrition preceding a new concep-tion.

Professor Geoffrey Chamberlain, an eminent obstetrician, conclud-ed from a survey of British births that the optimum interval between births is between two and four years.

Difficulty in conceiving

Most people take their fertility for granted, and a couple who decide to have a baby may be surprised when several months pass without a conception. Difficulty in conceiving has many possible causes and is more common than is generally perceived, with one-in-ten cou-ples failing to conceive within a year of planning to start a family.

Infertility is commonly attributed to the woman, although male fac-tors account for one-third of all infertility (Chamberlain, 1990). In general, the causes of infertility are thought to be approximately one-third male, one-third female and one-third couple-related.

Ninety per cent of couples having intercourse without using contra-ception will conceive within 18 months; the remaining 10 per cent are said to be sub-fertile. This does not mean they will never be able to have a child together, but medical investigation of the problem should be sought, since about 50 per cent of couples who do so eventually conceive.

In the meantime, because it can often take many months to see a specialist, there are some self-help methods you may like to consid-er including the use of an ovulation temperature planner kit, which is available at most chemists. This planner will help you predict when you are at your most fertile time of your menstrual cycle. The normal recommendation to couples trying to conceive is to 'save up sperm' by having intercourse every other day around this fertile time (time of expected ovulation). However, a report in the Lancet suggests that while this advice is appropriate for men who have a normal output of sperm, for men with a low output of healthy sperm, frequent intercourse is likely to increase sperm counts and fertility potential. The report therefore recommended that men diagnosed as having low sperm counts, may increase their chances of fertilisation by having intercourse every day or even twice a day at the time of ovulation.

For conception to take place several conditions must be fulfilled. As well as her partner's sperm count being healthy – the woman must be ovulating, her fallopian tubes must allow clear passage for the egg from the ovary to the uterus, and the sperm must be deposited close to the cervix at the time of the menstrual cycle when the egg has been released.

Some infertility arises from anatomical problems such as blocked fallopian tubes or fibroids, which may require surgical intervention. Medical and environmental factors which may influence ability to conceive include infection (the most common preventable cause of infertility in both men and women), frequency of menstrual cycle, age (peak fertility occurs between 20–25 years), physical health, drugs, smoking, alcohol and exposure to toxic substances.

The influence of nutrition

If a woman has a low body weight for her height, her chances of conceiving a baby are reduced.

Amenorrhoea (absence of periods) and infertility caused by food shortages are well known. Following the defeat of the German armies in the Second World War, food supplies were severely curtailed throughout Germany and, as a result, there was a 70 per cent fall in birth-rate in Frankfurt in 1944–45. The reduction in fertility was accompanied by an epidemic of infant deaths and birth abnormalities among babies conceived by women who remained fertile.

The mechanism by which nutrition affects fertility is probably through the endocrine or hormone system. The increase of infertility during food shortages suggests that the endocrine system is sensitive to nutritional status. It would appear that there is a nutritional infertility threshold, below which the endocrine system reduces secretion of reproductive hormones and women become infertile.

Similar findings occur with women suffering from the eating disorder, anorexia nervosa. When a woman continues to follow a strict regime which causes her to lose weight excessively, she will eventually become infertile.

OBSTETRIC HISTORY

Recommendation

A London teaching hospital study showed that underweight women who were prescribed drugs to promote ovulation (fertility drugs) had a high risk (54 per cent) of having a growth-retarded baby. The authors concluded that the most suitable treatment for infertility for those who were underweight and were not having regular periods was a dietary one, rather than inducing ovulation by pharmaceutical means (Van der Spuy, 1988). It is therefore wise to put off attempting to conceive for at least three or four months on a good diet following recovery from amenorrhoea.

Miscarriage

A pregnancy that ends spontaneously before 28 weeks of pregnancy is termed a miscarriage. It is estimated that miscarriage affects one woman in four. The feeling of loss can lead to intense feelings of bereavement and isolation. Women suffering from these emotions often feel dismissed by the medical profession. This may be because doctors themselves are often unable to explain why miscarriage happens in many cases.

The underlying causes of this distressing event can be identified in about 50 per cent of couples who suffer a miscarriage. Two common causes that can be investigated are cervical incompetence (weakness) and structural irregularities such as a fibroid in the womb. Miscarriage may also occur as the result of low hormone levels or hormonal imbalances, ectopic pregnancies or chromosomal disorders. The chances of having a miscarriage are increased for women who smoke or drink alcohol.

Much work has been carried out on human sperm and it is known that sperm abnormalities increase the risk of miscarriage. It is estimated that about half the miscarriages that occur are attributable to the male partner.

Particularly sad is the situation of women who have had repeated miscarriages. However, they should not lose hope, as statistics show that for a woman who has had two consecutive miscarriages the odds are that about one-third of future pregnancies may miscarry (Chamberlain, 1990). This still leaves two-thirds of pregnancies likely to result in the delivery of a normal healthy baby. Furthermore, the odds do not deteriorate greatly even after five miscarriages. Although each loss is an individual tragedy, 70 to 80 per cent of couples with a history of recurrent miscarriages eventually have a successful pregnancy (Cefalo and Moos, 1988). Many women who have persisted after so many disappointments have been happily rewarded for their perseverance.

Good pre-pregnancy health habits practised by both partners will contribute to a successful outcome of a future pregnancy. These include stopping smoking, healthy eating, target weight achievement, taking the recommended folic acid supplement and a low intake of alcohol and coffee and other caffeine-containing drinks.

Most importantly, you must give yourself time to recover both physically and emotionally. It is understandable that after such a disappointment, you would want to try again as soon as possible; but the physical health of both parents in the three months prior to conception can influence the health of both the sperm and the egg. Sperm can be stored in the male for up to three months and, if the miscarriage was the result of damaged sperm, time should be allowed for the quality to be restored.

The Miscarriage Association gives support and advice to women and their families during and after miscarriage. Their address is c/o Clayton Hospital, Northgate, Wakefield, W Yorkshire, WF1 3JS; telephone 01924 200799.

8

YOU AND YOUR PARTNER

The health of a father-to-be at the time of conception is now thought to be more important than previously acknowledged, and some experts believe that the father may share equal responsibility for an unfavourable pregnancy outcome such as miscarriage, premature birth and low birthweight, as well as congenital abnormalities.

However, attaching blame to one or other partner is not a constructive philosophy, but the premise of shared responsibility is. There may be biological limits to a father's influence on the outcome of pregnancy, but there are no limits to the ways in which he can support his partner. This help can include, for example, governing his smoking, his alcohol intake and improving his diet, while encouraging his partner to do the same. In helping in this way, he will make a very valuable contribution towards attaining good pre-pregnancy health practices and may also have a positive impact on his spermatogenesis and fertility.

There are a number of environmental and lifestyle factors which can cause damage to sperm. These include smoking, alcohol, drugs and exposure to radiation and to some chemicals. Nutrient deficiencies such as zinc and vitamin A have also been catalogued as having possible detrimental effects on spermatogenesis. However, the extent to which diet is implicated in male fertility remains unclear.

Smoking

Men who smoke have a much higher proportion of abnormal sperm than non-smokers. An increase in sperm abnormalities effectively reduces the sperm count, and preliminary evidence suggests that smoking may affect male fertility by altering spermatogenesis, sperm density, sperm motility and sperm morphology (Lincoln, 1986).

The evidence is incomplete as to the extent of the consequences of exposure of the mother to tobacco smoke, but overall, the effects do consistently suggest a detrimental influence on pregnancy outcome. The underlying mechanism by which these influences occur are not yet understood and more research needs to be undertaken in this area.

According to a large American study of non-smoking women whose partners smoked, the incidence of malformations in their babies increased significantly if fathers smoked more than ten cigarettes a day; the incidence of facial malformations was particularly influenced by number of cigarettes smoked. Other studies have not associated passive smoking with birth abnormalities but with an increase in the rate of low birthweight and the rate of premature births. (Nakamura M et al., 1987). Yet another study, this time in Germany, found that smoking by the father, when the mother did not smoke, was associated with an increased incidence of miscarriage, pre-term births and low birthweight (Koller, 1983).

Alcohol

Excessive alcohol may also affect the quality and quantity of sperm so it is wise for both partners to restrict their alcohol intake when trying to conceive.

Observations of a relationship between excess paternal drinking and reduced birthweight have been reported. One study showed a strong correlation between a father's alcohol intake in the month prior to conception and the infant's birthweight. This association was independent of the mother's alcohol intake. Another study reported that men who drink more than 30 ml of pure alcohol a day, equivalent to two pints of lager, fathered children who weighed, on average, 6 oz less than those fathers who drank less than that.

It has been found that the slight excess of male infants usually seen in the normal population is reduced in families where the father's occupation involves alcohol. Theoretically, this could be induced by lower testosterone in men who are heavy drinkers. Any reduction of testosterone levels not only reduces the man's libido but also his sperm count and function.

Nutrition

The testes, like the ovaries, are dependent for their function on the secretion of reproductive hormones which are influenced by nutrition.

Adequate vitamin C levels are needed for normal production of sperm. It is known that low blood vitamin C levels are associated with lower sperm count together with poor sperm quality and vitamin C supplementation leads to improvements in these characteristics.

Cigarette smoking is associated with low blood vitamin C levels and with reduced sperm count and increased rates of sperm abnormalities. Many studies on the effect of vitamin C supplementation on sperm quality of smokers showed that doses of 200 mg a day led to improvements in sperm quality in heavy smokers (Dawson et al., 1992).

Further improvements in sperm quality resulted from work by Takarhara et al. (1982) who reported reduced fertility in male patients with seminal zinc levels below 15 mg/dl. They found zinc supplementation effective in improving fertility in 50 per cent of cases.

Essential fatty acids (linoleic acid), vitamin A, vitamin E and zinc have all been reported to be essential for normal formation of sperm in animals. However few studies have been done on the effects of nutritional status of the human male and reproductive health and much more research is required in this area.

—— Family history – genetics ——

Genetics is a subject which claims our attention not just scientifically but also in a general sense. Most families can tell you about some physical feature or characteristic trait that keeps turning up from one generation to the next. It may be a cleft chin or red hair; it may be diabetes or cystic fibrosis or it may be that they all survive to a healthy, ripe old age. Skills such as football, car racing and golf often appear to pass from one generation to the next. Genetics is however, a random activity as George Bernard Shaw's aphorism underlines – when a famous actress suggested that with *his* brain and *her* looks, their child would be a force to be reckoned with,'Yes Madam,' he said, 'but what if hc has *my* looks and *your* brain?'

More serious are genetic diseases that can potentially be passed on from one generation to the next within families. There are different types of genetic diseases with varying risks of recurrence. For anyone with a family history of a genetically related disorder, it is usual for their doctor to refer them to a genetic counsellor who can carry out tests and calculate the risks of their having a baby with the disease for which they are carriers. They will also be told about the likely severity of the disease and whether there is any treatment available and any other information they need in order to make a decision.

One of the purposes of genetic counselling is to define risks and it is important to fully understand what is meant when told, for example, that there is a one-in-three chance of recurrence of an inherited disease. In such a situation it is sometimes interpreted that the two pregnancies following a pregnancy with such an outcome will be normal. A crucial principle relating to risk factors is that 'chance' does not have a memory. What is meant is that in *each* pregnancy there is a risk of one-in-three that the baby will be affected, not that out of three children, one will be affected.

Advances in antenatal diagnosis make it possible for some inherited diseases to be diagnosed early in pregnancy. This may be done either by a triple blood test which can be taken at 12 weeks of pregnancy or by taking and analysing some of the fluid surrounding the baby (amniocentesis). The latter is usually done at about 18 weeks and carries with it a small (two per cent) risk of miscarriage. The preferred method is now by the triple blood test which has the added advantages of earlier detection to allay any unwarranted concerns and no interference with the womb environment. If the fetus is affected, the parents have the option of having a therapeutic abortion; if all is well, they will have peace of mind to enjoy the remainder of the pregnancy.

9

SOME MYTHS AND
SOME NOT

As soon as you become pregnant, you will probably be bombarded with all sorts of advice on pregnancy from family members and friends, some of which may be sound and scientifically accurate, and some of which may be classed as benign 'old wives tales' or folklore. An attempt is made here to discuss some of the more common misunderstandings.

True or false?

Can the sex of the baby be influenced by food choice and other means?

Girls are made of sugar and spice
and all things nice
Boys are made of frogs and snails
and puppy dogs tails

Wanting to have a child of a particular sex is a normal desire. It appears that most couples tend to have a preference for the first born to be a male child. Unfortunately in many cultures this apparently harmless preference has resulted in positive rejection of female children. However, there can be good reasons for seeking a child of a particular gender where, because of inherited illnesses which can continue through one or other of the sexes.

Attempts at sex determination at childbirth has been with us since time began. Folklore suggested that sexual selection could be obtained in some very obscure ways such as sexual positions during intercourse or bandaging of one testicle or other to produce the desired sex.

One basic fact is known – it is the father who determines the sex of the baby. Both partners have 23 pairs of chromosomes, having received half from each parent. These chromosomes determine the baby's inherited characteristics. Each chromosome carries about 2,000 genes, and it is the genes which determine such things as the baby's sex, hair and eye colour, height, build and blood group. The genes also influence traits such as intelligence and personality but these will also be affected by other factors such as the environment in which the child is brought up.

One pair, the sex chromosomes, consist of X and Y chromosomes. A normal female has two X chromosomes and a normal male will have an X and Y chromosome. The female ovum or egg can therefore only contain an X while the male sperm cell can carry an X or Y. If the fertilising sperm contains an X chromosome, the baby will be a girl and if it contains a Y chromosome, the baby will be a boy. The timing of sexual determination is at the moment of conception and nothing can alter that at a later date. For most couples, the chances of a boy or girl are approximately equal but the laws of probability are such that a minority of families will have all boys and some will have all girls.

Numerous ways of influencing the desired sex of a child have been advocated but none of them are effective or stand up to scientific scrutiny.

Some have suggested that the acidity of the woman's vagina may favour X-bearing sperm, so it is thought that a gel with an acid base introduced into the vagina will favour male-making sperm.

Others have speculated that the sex of baby can be influenced by the parents eating certain foods before conception. Publicity has been given to some work that advises women who want a boy to eat foods high in salt and potassium but low in calcium and magnesium. Conversely, couples who want to have a daughter should eat a diet high in calcium and magnesium and low in sodium and potassium. Although the advice focuses on women, who it is suggested should start this regime six weeks prior to conceiving, it recommended their partners should also go on the diet to give moral support. The rationale for this advice is that the surface of the egg will be more receptive to fertilisation by sperm of the chosen sex.

Although a high rate of success is claimed, there are no medical grounds to support it.

'Boy Foods'	'Girl Foods'
Foods that are:	Foods that are:
High salt, high potassium	High calcium, high magnesium
Low calcium, low magnesium	Low salt, low potassium

Caution should be exercised as there is no scientific justification that diet intervention prior to pregnancy affects gender outcome and restriction of any group of nutrients, particularly calcium and magnesium, is contrary to the general advice given in this book.

True or false?

The baby will always get enough nutrition, no matter what the mother eats.

The concept that the fetus is a parasite was based on the assumption that the metabolic rate of the fetus was much faster than that of the mother. This should allow the fetus to compete favourably for available nutrients. However the issue is a very complex one. If the mother is undernourished, the growth of the placenta is likely to be reduced so that the capacity of the placenta to transport nutrients to the fetus may be diminished. There is no clear cut answer, but in general, the placenta will concentrate most vitamins to the benefit of the fetus but this is not the case for all nutrients.

True or false?

During pregnancy you need to eat for two.

Stores of vitamins and minerals are thought to be utilised during pregnancy. This may be difficult if stores are low at the start of pregnancy but the body stimulates adaptive responses such as increased ability to absorb some nutrients such as iron and calcium and reduce urinary excretion of other nutrients such as vitamin B2. These responses help meet the increased demands for nutrients, irrespective of the nutritional status of the mother.

True or false?

Hair analysis is a good method of assessing your nutritional status for pregnancy.

Hair analysis as a means of detecting nutritional deficiencies remains a controversial issue. The consensus is that tests on blood and urine are better indicators of nutritional status. Proponents of hair analysis argue that sophisticated laboratory equipment allows great accuracy in hair analysis. While this may be true, the results of hair analyses do not necessarily reflect amounts of nutrients found in the tissues and there are large variations in what are considered normal concentrations depending on age, hair colour and even the part of the head from which the hair is taken.

True or false?

Stout is good for pregnant women because it contains iron.

Stout does contain some vitamins and minerals but the amounts are too small to be of any nutritional significance – half a pint of stout will provide 0.14 mg of iron, less than 1 per cent of the recommended daily intake (14.8 mg). It does however contain alcohol which is not really recommended for either partner when trying to conceive.

True or false?

If the mother's diet is deficient she will crave the food that contains the nutrient that she is lacking.

Some mothers do experience food cravings during their pregnancy. These cravings can vary from foods such as pickled onions to unusual combinations of foods, all of which usually bear little relationship to nutrient deficiencies.

Although unusual in this country, some women may have cravings for non-foods and practice *pica*. Pica is a compulsion to eat substances of little or no nutritional value such as clay, chalk, laundry starch, burnt matches or ice. Practising pica can interfere with the absorption of essential nutrients, for example clay inhibits the absorption of iron.

True or false?

Children born in the autumn do better at school than children born in summer.

Local authorities have been looking at performance at GCSEs and have consistently found that the best achievers were born between September and December, the difference equating to two GCSE grades. This is thought to be due to the autumn born children having a two-term advantage over the summer born children, the effects of which seem to continue long after primary school age. So, no nutritional claims are made here, but you may like to consider the timing of your planned pregnancy to coincide with an autumn baby!

True or false?

Drink during pregnancy can create murderers.

This rather alarming statement appeared as the heading of a piece in *The Times* in June 1993. A third of the inmates on Death Row in the USA, it suggested, suffered from fetal-alcohol syndrome in which alcohol interfered at a critical stage of brain development which occurs in the early stages of pregnancy. This, according to some, is when the nerve cells start making connections and, if the process does not happen at that time, it will never happen. The headline was of course less than honest in that here we are talking about someone who drinks very heavily. None the less, until a 'safe' limit is determined, the advice must continue to be to abstain from alcohol if you are trying to have a baby.

True or false?

Men who eat organic food are twice as fertile as those who do not.

There has been a dramatic decline in male fertility over the past 50 years. Studies in over 20 countries show that men are producing only half the number of sperm as the average man did in the 1930s, a change which some scientists attribute to chemicals in the food chain.

A Danish study tested the sperm density (number of sperm per ml of semen) and sperm count (number of active sperm per million) of organic farmers. These farmers ate a high proportion of pesticide-free home-grown food and organic dairy products. The study found their sperm density and sperm count was almost twice as high as those of a group of printers, electricians and metal workers. Their sperm count was also much higher. While this may be true for that particular population, it was a small study and the results need to be substantiated with larger numbers in different populations.

True or false?

Pregnancy improves the health of the hair but childbirth makes your hair fall out.

During pregnancy the normal hair-shedding mechanism is slowed down, probably because of the high oestrogen levels in the woman's blood. After giving birth her hormone levels change, and the hair that she would have shed gradually, is shed much more quickly.

True or false?

VDUs (visual display units) can harm unborn babies.

There has been some concern about reports of a higher incidence of miscarriages and birth defects among VDU users. Many studies have been carried out which, overall, do not show any link between miscarriages or birth defects and working with VDUs.

True or false?

The mother should only gain the weight of the baby i.e. 6–9 lb.

The mother has to gain more than the weight of the baby. The extra weight gained will be accounted for by the placenta, increase in maternal blood volume, amniotic fluid which surrounds and protects the unborn baby and extra fat which is laid down in preparation for breast feeding. A woman of normal weight should gain between 20 and 30 lb for pregnancy. Poor weight gain is associated with low-birthweight infants.

True or false?

If you take a multivitamin pill you don't need to worry about eating well.

There is no reason why you should not take a multivitamin or mineral supplement but this will not provide the protein, essential fatty acids, fibre or energy that you also need for a 'complete' diet. In any case, the majority of supplements do not supply every vitamin or mineral that is essential to health so it would be unwise to suppose you had a comprehensive insurance against deficits in your diet (see page 49 on supplementation).

True or false?

It is unwise to exercise during pregnancy.

Although vigorous exercise should be discouraged during the third trimester of pregnancy, a pregnant woman can continue with her normal exercise routine with no ill effects to her unborn baby. It is not however recommended to suddenly start demanding exercise regimes when pregnant. Swimming, moderate levels of exercise such as walking or cycling will help you get/stay fit. Exercise also relieves stress. Being physically fit during pregnancy can help ease labour, and help you to return to your pre-pregnancy weight more quickly.

True or false?

The woman never gets back to her original weight once she's had a baby.

Some women do have a hard time getting back to their pre-pregnancy weight, but often these are the women who lead sedentary lifestyles. Women who take regular exercise prior to and during pregnancy can usually get back to their original weight without much difficulty.

True or false?

The stomach's high or low profile indicates the sex of the unborn child.

There is no evidence to substantiate the claim. The stomach's profile is irrelevant to the sex of the unborn child.

APPENDIX 1

A summary of advice

Department of Health advice

- Take a 400 mcg supplement of folic acid every day if you are planning or are likely to become pregnant. This should be continued for 8 to 12 weeks after you conceive.
- Avoid liver or liver products because of the exceptionally high vitamin A content.

Bad habits

- Cut out smoking
- Drink alcohol moderately or not at all
- Avoid non-essential drugs.

Healthy eating

- Enjoy food!
- Have three meals a day
- Have each day:

    Bread, cereals and starchy foods – 4 to 5 portions
    Vegetables – at least 2 portions
    Fruit – at least 2 portions
    Meat, fish, eggs and pulses – 2 portions
    Milk, cheese and yogurt – 2 portions

- High sugar, high fat foods – have them 'occasionally'.

Safety with food

- Follow the advice on food safety and hygiene in Chapter 4.

Safety with pets

- Follow the advice about hygiene with pets, especially with cats, in Chapter 4.

Health problems

- Sort out any health problems you have. If in doubt, seek advice from your doctor.

Birth Spacing

- Allow two years between births.

APPENDIX 2

—— Body Mass Index ——

HEIGHT (Feet and Inches)

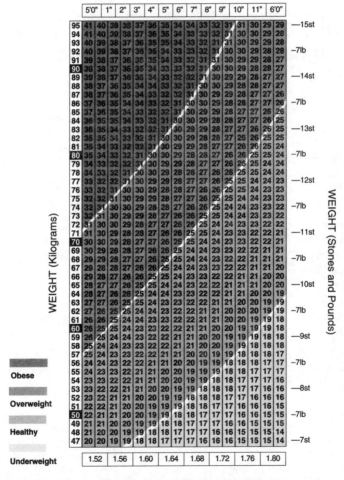

WEIGHT (Kilograms)

WEIGHT (Stones and Pounds)

Obese

Overweight

Healthy

Underweight

Adapted from Garrow JS 1981, Churchill Livingstone, England

APPENDIX 3

Daily Dietary Requirements for non--pregnant women and women during-pregnancy (DoH, 1991)

		Non-pregnant women 19–50 yrs	Increment for pregnancy
Energy	kcals	1940	+200**
Protein	g	45	+6
Fibre	g	18	*
Vitamins			
Thiamin (B1)	mg	0.8	+0.1
Riboflavin (B2)	mg	1.1	+0.3
Niacin (B3)	mg	13	*
Vitamin B6	mg	1.2	*
Folic acid	mcg	200	+400 ***
Vitamin A	mcg	600	+100
Vitamin C	mg	40	+10
Vitamin D	mcg	–	10
Minerals			
Calcium	mg	700	*
Iron	mg	14.8	*
Magnesium	mg	270	*
Zinc	mg	7	*

* no increment
** for last trimester only
*** preconceptionally and until 12th week of pregnancy

APPENDIX 4

---------- **References** ----------

Chapter 1

Barker, D.J.P., Gluckman, P.D., Godfrey, K.M., Harding, J.E., Owens, J.A. and Robinson, J.S. (1993) Fetal nutrition and cardiovascular disease in adult life. *Lancet*, 341: 938–941

Eckhert, C.D. and Hurley, L.S. (1977) Reduced DNA synthesis in zinc deficiency: regional differences in embryonic rats. *J. Nutr.* 107: 855–61

Fedrick, J. and Adelstein, P. (1978) Factors associated with low birthweight of infants delivered at term. *Br. J. Obstet. & Gyn.* 85(1): 1–7

Institute of Medicine. (1985) *Preventing Low Birthweight.* National Academy Press: Washington

Metcoff, J.A. et al. (1981) Maternal nutrition and fetal outcome. *Am. J. Clin Nutr.* 34: 708–721

Office of Populations, Censuses and Surveys. (1988) *Congenital malformation statistics 1981–85: notifications.* Series MB3 no 2, HMSO: London

Pharoah, P.O.D., Cooke, T., Cooke, R.W.I. and Rosenbloom, L. (1990) Birthweight specific trends in cerebral palsy. *Arch. of Dis. in Childhood,* (65) 602–606

Pirke, K.M., Schweiger, U., Lemmel, W., Krieg, J.C. and Berger, M. (1985) The influence of dieting on the menstrual cycle of healthy young women. *J. Clin. Endocrinol. Metab.* 60: 1174–9

Scottish Low Birthweight Study Group (1992) The Scottish low birthweight study: I. Survival, neurometer and sensory impairment. *Arch. of Disease in Childhood.* 67: 675–681

Sutherland, H. (1981) Letter to the Editor. The *Lancet*, 1

World Health Organisation (1980) The incidence of low birthweight; a critical review of available information. *World Health Stats. Quart.* 33: 197–214

Chapter 2

British Nutrition's Task Force Report (1992) *Unsaturated fatty acids – nutritional and physiological significance*. Chapman and Hall

Ceizel, A.E. (1993) Prevention of congenital abnormalities by periconceptional multivitamin supplementation. B.M.J., 306: 1645–1648

Department of Health (1990) PL/CMO(90)11

Department of Health (1991) Dietary Reference Values for Food Energy and Nutrients for the UK. *COMA Report on Health & Social Subjects No 41.* HMSO: London

Department of Health (1992) *Folic Acid and the Prevention of Neural Tube Defects*

Doyle, W., Crawford, M.A., Wynn, A.H.A. and Wynn, S.W. (1990) The association between maternal diet and birth dimensions. *J. Nutr. Med.* 1: 9–17

Doyle, W., Wynn, A.H.A., Crawford, M.A. and Wynn, S.W. (1992) Nutritional counselling and supplements in the second and third trimester of pregnancy, a study in a London population. *J. Nutr. Med.* 3: 249–56

Gregory, J., Foster, K., Taylor, H. and Wiseman, M. (1990) *The Dietary and Nutritional Survey of British Adults*. HMSO: London

Hurley, L.S. and Mutch, P.B. (1973) Prenatal and postnatal development after transitory gestational zinc deficiency in rats. *J. Nutrition*, 103: 649–656

Institute of Medicine (1990) *Nutrition During Pregnancy*. Washington: National Academy Press.

Jameson, S. (1976) Effects of zinc deficiency in human reproduction. *Acta Med. Scand. (Suppl.)*, 593:1–89

Kitay, D.Z. and Habort, R.A. (1975) Iron and folic acid deficiency in pregnancy. *Clin. Perinatol.* 2: 255

Purdie, D.W. (1989) Bone metabolism and reproduction. *Contemporary Reviews in Obs. & Gynae.* 1: 214–221

Reeve, J. (1991) Calcium metabolism. In: Hytten F. and Chamberlain G.V.P. (eds). *Clinical Physiology in Obstetrics*. Second edition. Oxford: Blackwell Scientific Publications

Saunders, T.A.B. and Reddy, S. (1994) Nutritional implications of a meatless diet. *Proc. Nutr. Soc.* 53: 297–307

Van Gelder, D.W. and Darby, F.V. (1944) Congenital and infantile beriberi. *J. Pediatr.* 25: 226–235

Wald, N., Sneddon, J., Densem, J., Frost, C. and Stone, R. (1991) Prevention of neural tube defects: results of the Medical Research Council Vitamin Study. *Lancet*, 338: 131–137

Wynn, A.H.A., Crawford, M.A., Doyle, W. and Wynn, S.W. (1991) Nutrition of women in anticipation of pregnancy. *Nutr. & Health*, 7: 69–88

Chapter 3

Department of Health. Dietary Reference Values for Food Energy and Nutrients for the UK. COMA Report on Health & Social Subjects No 41. HMSO, London, 1991

Department of Health. (1992) *Folic Acid and the Prevention of Neural Tube Defects*

Doyle, W., Crawford, M.A., Wynn, A.H.A. and Wynn, S.W. (1990) The association between maternal diet and birth dimensions. *J. Nutr. Med.* 1: 9–17

Wynn, A.H.A., Crawford, M.A., Doyle, W. and Wynn, S.W. (1991) Nutrition of women in anticipation of pregnancy. *Nutr. & Health*, 7: 69–88

Chapter 4

Department of Health. (1992) *While you are pregnant: Safe eating and how to avoid infection from food and animals*. HMSO. O/N 19912 HSSH J1560NE

Crawford, M.A., Doyle, W., Drury, P., Lennon, A., Costello, K. and Leighfield, M. (1989) n-6 and n-3 fatty acids during early human development. *Jrnl. of Internal Medicine.* Vol 225, Suppl 1: 159–169

Doyle, W., Crawford, M.A., Wynn, A.H.A. and Wynn, S.W. (1990) The association between maternal diet and birth dimensions. *J. Nutr. Med.* 1: 9–17

Doyle, W., Jenkins, S., Crawford, M.A. and Puvandendran, K. (1994) The Nutritional status of school children in an inner city area. *Arch. of Dis. in Childhood*, 70: 376–381

Olsen, S.F., Hansen, H.S., Sorensen, T.I.A. et al. (1986) Intake of marine fat, rich in (n-3)-polyunsaturated fatty acids, may increase birthweight by prolonged gestation. *Lancet*, 367–369

Chapter 5

Bernstein, L., Pike, M., Lobo, R., Depue, R.H., Ross, R.K. and Henderson, B.E. (1989) Cigarette smoking in pregnancy results in marked decrease in hCG and oestradiol levels. *Br. J. Obst. & Gyn.* 96: 92–96

Brooke, O.G., Anderson, H.R., Bland, J.M., Peacock, J.L. and Stewart, C.M. (1989) Effects on birthweight of smoking, alcohol, caffeine, socioeconomic factors, and psychosocial stress. *Br. Med. J.* 298: 795–801

Bullard, J.A. (1981) Exercise and pregnancy. *Can. Fam. Physician,* 27: 977–982

Chamberlain, G. (1990) *Preparing for pregnancy.* Fontana Paperbacks: London

Field, B. and Kerr, C. (1981). Season and interval of recurrence of neural tube defects. *Jnl. of Med. Genetics,* 18: 484.

Fogelman, K.R. and Manor, O. (1988) Smoking in pregnancy and development into early adulthood. *Br. Med. J.* 297: 1233–1236

Elwood, P.C. et al. (1987) Growth of children from 0–5 years: with special reference to mother's smoking in pregnancy. *Annals of Human Biology,* 14, 6: 543–557

Infante-Rivarde, C., Fernandez, A., Gauthier, R., David, M., Rivard, G.E. (1993) Fetal loss associated with caffeine intake before and during pregnancy. *Jnl. Am. Med. Ass.* 270(24): 2940–3

Khoury, M.J., Gomez-Faria, M. and Mulinare, J. (1989) Does maternal cigarette smoking during pregnancy cause cleft lip and palate in offspring? *Am. J. Dis. of Childhood,* 143: 333–337

Koller, S. (1983) *Pisikofaktoren der Schwangerschaft.* Heidelberg: Springer-Verlag

Lincoln, R. (1986) Smoking and reproduction. *Fam. Planning Perspect.* 18: 79–84

Mills, J.L., Graubard, B.I., Harley, E.E., Rhoads, G.G. and Berendes, H.W. (1984) Maternal alcohol consumption and birthweight: how much drinking during pregnancy is safe? *J.A.M.A.* 252: 1875–1879

Mosher, W.D. and Pratt, W.F. (1987) Reproductive impairment in married couples. *United States Vital and Health Statistics: National Survey of Family Growth,* Series 23, No 11

Newspeil, D.R., Rush, D., Butler, N.R., Golding, J., Bijur, P.E. and Kurzon,

M. (1989) Parental smoking and post-infancy wheezing in children: a prospective cohort study. *Am. J. Public Health*, 79: 168–171

Rosevear, S.K., Holt, D.W., Lee, T.D., Ford, W.C.L., Wardle, P.G. and Hull, M.G.R. (1992) Smoking and decreased fertilisation rates in-vitro. *Lancet*, 340: 1195–96

Sulaiman, N.D. et al. (1988) Alcohol consumption in Dundee, Primagravida and its effects on outcome of pregnancy. *B. Med. J.*, May, 1988

Chapter 6

Bates, G.W., Bates, S.W. and Whitworth, N.S. (1982) Reproductive failure in women who practise weight control. *Fertility & Sterility*, 37: 3, 373–378

Beasley, R.P., Hwang, L.Y., Lee, G.C. et al. (1983) Prevention of perinatally transmitted hepatitis B virus infections with hepatitis B immune globulin and hepatitis B vaccine. *Lancet*, 2: 1099–1102

Ho-Yen, D.O. and Joss, A.W.L. (1988) Toxoplasma and cytomegalovirus infections during pregnancy. *Matern. Child Health*, 13: 225–7

Hurley, R. (1983) Virus infection in pregnancy and the puerperium. *Recent Advances in Clinical Virology*. Ed. A.P. Waterson. Churchill-Livingstone

Reid, T.M.S. (1990) Infections. In: *Perspectives in Pre-pregnancy Counselling*. Eds. H.W. Sutherland & N.C. Smith. Smith-Gordon & Co. Ltd

Van der Spuy, Z.M., Steer, P.J., McCusker, M., Steele, S.J., Jacobs, H.S. (1988) Outcome of pregnancy in underweight women after spontaneous and induced ovulation. *Br. Med. J.* 296: 962–965

Wang, E. and Smaill F. (1989) *The Guide to Effective Care in Pregnancy and Childbirth*. Ed. Enkin, M., Keirse, M.J.N.C., Chalmers, I. Oxford: Oxford University Press

Wynn, A. & Wynn, M. (1990) The need for nutritional assessment in the treatment of the infertile patient. *J. Nutr. Med.* 1: 315–324

Chapter 7

Bates, G.W., Bates, S.W. and Whitworth, N.S. (1982) Reproductive failure in women who practise weight control. *Fertility & Sterility*, 37: 3, 373–378

Cefalo, R.C. and Moos, Merry-K. (1988) *Preconceptional Health Promotion, A Practical Guide*. Aspen Publishers

Chamberlain, G. (1990) *Preparing for Pregnancy*. London: Fontana Paperbacks

Chamberlain, G., Philipp, E., Howlett, B. and Claireaux, A. (1975) British Births 1970. 2: *Obstetric Care*. London: Heinemann.

Chanarin, I. (1979) Distribution of folate deficiency. In Botez, M.I. and Reynolds, E.H. (Eds) *Folic Acid in Neurology, Psychiatry and Internal Medicine*. New York: Raven Press

Martin, E.C. (1978) Birth intervals and development of nine-year-olds in Singapore. *I.P.P.F. Medical Bulletin*, 12: No 3, 1–3

Mosher, W.D., Pratt, W.F. (1987) Reproductive impairment in married couples. *United States Vital and Health Statistics: National Survey of Family Growth*, Series 23, No 11. Publication PHS 83-1987. Washington, DC, US Public Health Service

Van der Spuy, Z.M., Steer, P.J., McCusker, M., Steele, S.J., Jacobs, H.S. (1988) Outcome of pregnancy in underweight women after spontaneous and induced ovulation. *Br. Med. J.* 296: 962–965

Worthington-Roberts, B. and Rodwell-Williams, S. (1989) *Nutrition in Pregnancy and Lactation*. Times Mirror/Mosby College Publ. 1989

Wynn, A. (1987) Nutrition before conception and the outcome of pregnancy. *Nutr. & Health* 5: No 1/2 31–43

Chapter 8

Chamberlain, G. (1990) *Preparing for pregnancy*. London: Fontana Paperbacks

Dawson, Earl B. et al. (1992) Effect of ascorbic acid supplementation on the sperm quality of smokers. *Fertility & Sterility*, 58(5): 1034–1039

Koller, S. (1983) *Pisikofaktoren der Schwangerschaft*, Heidelberg: Springer-Verlag

Lincoln, R. (1986) Smoking and reproduction. *Fam. Planning Perspect.* 18: 79–84

Nakamura, M. et al. (1987) *Effect of passive smoking by husband on pregnancy outcomes – a population-based prospective study from Japan*, 6th World Conf. on Smoking & Health, Tokyo, Nov. 87

Takahara, H., Cosentino, M.J. and Cockett, A.T.K. (1982) Zinc therapy or in combination with varicocelectomy to improve the fertility potential of the male. *J. Androl.* 3: 37

APPENDIX 5

———— Useful addresses ————

The Association for Spina Bifida & Hydrocephalus
ASBAH House
Park Road
Peterborough PE1 2UQ
Tel. 01733 555988

The Cystic Fibrosis Research Trust
Alexander House
5 Blyth Road
Bromley
Kent BR1 3RS
Tel. 0181 464 7211

The Down's Syndrome Association
155 Mitcham Road
Tooting
London SW17 9PG
Tel. 0181 682 4001

The Family Planning Association
27 Mortimer Street
London W1N 7RJ
Helpline 0171 636 7866

The Miscarriage Association
c/o Clayton Hospital
Wakefield
West Yorkshire WF1 3JS
Tel. 01924 200799

The National Childbirth Trust
Alexandra House
Oldham Terrace
London W3 6NH
Tel. 0181 992 8637

SANDS
The Stillbirth and Neonatal Death Society
28 Portland Place
London W1N 4DE
Helpline 0171 436 5881

SAFTA
Support Around Termination for Abnormality
29–30 Soho Square
London W1V 6JB
Tel. 0171 439 6124

The Toxoplasmosis Trust
61–71 Collier Street
London N1 9BE
Tel. 0171 713 0599

Foresight
Association for the Promotion of Pre-Conceptual Care
28 The Paddock
Godalming
Surrey GU7 1XD
Tel. 01483 427839

For help to give up smoking

Written advice
Action on Smoking & Health
109 Gloucester Place
London W1H 3PH
Tel. 0171 935 3519

Counselling
Telephone **Quitline** on 0171 487 3000

GLOSSARY

Amenorrhoea   absence or abnormal cessation of menstrual cycle

Anaemia   (*an* = without, *aemia* = blood) a condition where there are too few mature red blood cells, or they contain too little haemoglobin, to carry enough oxygen to the tissues

Antenatal   (*ante* – before) before birth; the period between conception and birth

Autism   mental condition, especially in children, in which the sufferer appears to be very withdrawn and absorbed in their own thoughts, preventing them from responding to their surroundings

Cerebral palsy   a condition where brain damage causes spasticity and uncontrolled movements

Cervix   neck of the womb

Chromosome   a structure within every cell that carries genetic information which passes from parents to child

Complex carbohydrates   starchy, fibre-containing foods, including wholegrain cereals, bread, rice, pasta, potatoes, vegetables and fruit

Congenital   applies to conditions that exist at or before birth

Congenital abnormalities   structural deficiencies of organs and limbs which occur during fetal life, i.e. before the baby is born

Cytology   study of the cells of the body

Ectopic pregnancy   a rare but serious condition where implantation occurs outside the womb, usually in the fallopian tube

Embryo   a term used to describe the developing infant from the third week after conception to the end of the eighth week, by which time all the major organs are discernible. After that the unborn infant is referred to as a fetus

Fertilisation   impregnation of the female egg, the ovum, by the male sex cell, the sperm

Fetal   see fetus

Fetus   from week 9 after conception until birth, the developing infant is called a fetus. During fetal life, cell differentiation and growth of the organs formed during the embryonic phase, occurs

Fibroid   a benign (non-malignant) tumour of muscle and connective tissue, usually embedded in the wall of the uterus

Follicle   the small sac of fluid in which the immature egg matures. Around day fourteen of the menstrual cycle the egg is released from the follicle

Gene   a unit involved in the transmission of hereditary characteristics from parent to child

Genito-urinary   referring to both the reproductive organs and the urinary tract

Gestation   means pregnancy: Most commonly used when describing number of weeks or duration of pregnancy that have elapsed since the first day of the last normal period or menstruation

Gynaecologist   a medical doctor who specialises in the reproductive system of women

Haemoglobin   the red pigment in blood that carries oxygen around the body

Hormones   help to regulate chemical processes that go on in the body. They are generated in specific organs such as the thyroid gland. Thyroid hormones affect growth in children and they control the rate at which our bodies use up nutrients i.e. metabolic rate. Other hormones include: the sex hormones, testosterone, which stimulates sex characteristics in men, and oestrogen and progesterone in women; insulin which helps to regulate blood sugar levels; and adrenalin which prepares the body for action in stressful situations

Miscarriage   spontaneous loss of a baby occurring up to 24 weeks gestation; after 24 weeks, the loss is termed a stillbirth

Mutagenic   an agent that can cause a change in genetic material, causing a new characteristic to appear. Some agents such as tobacco, alcohol or other chemical compounds, may lead to cell damage and disease

Neural tube defects   a group of congenital malformations in the embryonic development of the brain, skull and spinal column. These are caused by failure of the embryo's neural tube, which houses the nervous system, to close properly. The three most common neural tube defects are spina bifida, anencephaly and encephalocele

Obstetrician   a medical doctor who specialises in pregnancy and childbirth

Oestrogen   one of the two major female hormones, made in the adrenal gland and the ovary. It is essential for the maintenance of pregnancy and to the growing fetus

Organogenesis   the time when the organs of the body are being formed. Organogenesis begins after the fertilised egg is implanted in the womb and is more or less complete at 8 weeks

Ovaries   two female reproductive organs in which the egg cells, the ova, are contained. At the time of birth the ovaries contain their full quota of egg cells

Ovum   an egg cell produced in the ovary

Perinatal   (*peri* = around, *natal* = birth) relating to the time around birth

Placenta   acts as the exchange station between a mother and her developing baby. It is a vascular structure supplying the fetus with nutrients and oxygen and carrying away waste material and carbon dioxide through the connecting umbilical cord

Pre-eclampsia   a disorder of pregnancy associated with high blood pressure, protein in the urine (albuminuria) and swelling, particularly of ankles

Premature delivery   birth occurs after 20 weeks and before 37 weeks of gestation

Progesterone   progesterone and oestrogen are the two most prominent female sex hormones. One of the major functions of progesterone is to maintain the state of pregnancy by suppressing contractions of the uterus

Rubella   another name for German measles

Sperm   the male sex cell produced in large quantities in seminal fluid or semen. Originates from a Greek word meaning seed

Spermatogenesis   refers to the entire sequence of events that transform primitive germ cells into sperm

Spina bifida   see neural tube defects

Teratogen   any agent or disease having the ability to cause abnormalities or deviations from normal fetal development

Term pregnancy   pregnancy in which the baby is delivered between 37 and 42 weeks

Trimester   a third of pregnancy in terms of time. The first trimester is considered to be 0 to 13 weeks; the second trimester 14 to 27 weeks; and 28 weeks to term, the third trimester.

Uterus   womb

Vascular   network of vessels for transporting blood around the body

Womb   organ in female mammals in which the developing fetus is nourished until birth

Zygote   the fertilised egg

INDEX